Families of
Schizophrenic Patients

Families of Schizophrenic Patients
Cognitive behavioural intervention

Christine Barrowclough

Consultant Clinical Psychologist
South Manchester Health Authority
UK
and

Nicholas Tarrier

Professor
Clinical Psychology and Behavioural Sciences
University of Manchester
and
Head of Department
Clinical Psychology
South Manchester Health Authority
UK

First published in 1992 by:
Chapman & Hall
Reprinted in 1997 by:
Stanley Thornes (Publishers) Ltd

Reprinted in 2001 by:
Nelson Thornes Ltd
Delta Place
27 Bath Road
CHELTENHAM
GL53 7TH
United Kingdom

Transferred to digital print on demand, 2006

A catalogue record for this book is available from the British Library

ISBN 978 0 7487 3502 0

Page make-up by Best-set Typesetter Ltd

Printed and bound by CPI Antony Rowe, Eastbourne

Contents

Contents

Acknowledgements

We are indebted to all the families who took part in the Salford Family Intervention Project, to our colleagues on that project: Kath Porceddu, J.S. Bamrah, Christine Vaughn, Hugh Freeman and Sue Watts, and to Max Birchwood and his colleagues for permission to print the Social Functioning Scale.

Introduction

Schizophrenia is probably the major mental health problem facing contemporary society. The emotional, social, and economic costs of the disorder are enormous. Approximately one in every 100 of the population world-wide will suffer from the illness, the onset of which is typically late adolescence and early adulthood. It is doubly distressing that the illness, which can be so emotionally and socially crippling, strikes at a time of life which is full of aspiration and hope. Finding that their expectations of the future are potentially in ruins can greatly compound the burden of the illness to the patient, and to his or her family and friends.

The last decade has seen the development of psychological methods for dealing with the symptoms and other consequences of schizophrenia. An important area has been the work with families and patients, which has demonstrated that the risk of relapse can be reduced and the quality of life of the sufferer and their relatives increased through psychosocial interventions.

This text describes a cognitive-behavioural approach to addressing the needs of schizophrenic patients and their families. The management methods described derive from a family intervention programme used in the Salford Family Intervention Project, a large-scale research study carried out in Salford District Health Authority, UK, between 1982–7. The Project was designed to evaluate the effectiveness of different interventions in reducing schizophrenic relapse, and in increasing the level of social functioning of the patient. As co-directors of the Project, the authors gained considerable clinical experience in working with families of schizophrenics.

As this book is not intended to be an academic text, a detailed and critical account of the research literature is not included. Rather, we have provided summaries of the literature where appropriate, to give the reader an adequate background knowledge of the relevant area. Further reading is suggested at the end of the book for those who wish to acquaint themselves in more detail with the literature.

As with all cognitive-behaviour therapy, the careful analysis of specific problems guides the nature of the selected interventions. In this way the interventions are assessment-driven. Throughout the practical guidelines for working with families, we continually emphasize the importance of a thorough and continued analysis.

Chapter 1 provides background information about the history of schizophrenia, diagnostic issues, symptoms, and the utility of the vulnerability-stress model for understanding relapse – the conceptualization of schizophrenia that underpins psychological management and treatment. This chapter provides a useful summary for those less familiar with the literature, as well as supplying explanations suitable for helping relatives to understand the illness.

Chapter 2 reviews the contribution of the measure of Expressed Emotion (EE) to our knowledge about the influence of environmental factors on the course of schizophrenia. EE is a dichotomous rating made from an audio-taped interview with the patient's relative. The majority of research studies have shown there is a significant association between returning to live with a relative rated as high EE and increased relapse rates. However, EE is essentially a research measure which is unsuitable for use in a service setting. Ways in which the measure can be used to generate clinically useful information are discussed; these issues are again raised in Chapter 4 in the context of assessment methods.

Chapter 3 reviews the major studies of the family management of schizophrenia. The results of family intervention studies are summarized, and the relative effectiveness of the components of the intervention are discussed. The primary measure of outcome in the intervention trials has been relapse, and the need for multiple outcome assessments is emphasized. These are especially important in a clinical service setting, where contact with the patient and his or her family may continue over a long period of time, and measures such as social functioning, quality of life, and burden of care may become more salient than simple relapse rates.

The next four chapters cover the practical considerations of how to carry out the interventions. Here we describe the principles behind the interventions, and show through case examples how these could be implemented. Throughout the book we have adopted the attitude that the best way to improve the management of schizophrenia is to have available a number of options and approaches to deal with the specific patient's problems. Intervention with the family, described in Chapters 4 to 7, represent a set of such options.

The needs of the family can be loosely divided into three areas: receiving information about schizophrenia, its consequences and its management; acquiring the skills with which to manage stress; and being able to encourage and facilitate increased levels of functioning. A variety of assessment approaches are described in Chapter 4, providing the basis with which to address the problems of meeting these needs through various intervention options. Chapter 5 discusses the various issues around providing the family with information about schizophrenia. (Appendices 5 and 6 include information that can be given to families, and an interview schedule (KASI) for assessing the knowledge the relative has about schizophrenia.)

Chapter 6 addresses the topic of managing and coping with the stress of caring for someone suffering a severe mental illness, and how these coping skills can be facilitated. Chapter 7 deals with the contructional approach to coping with problems and difficulties, and how increases in levels of functioning can be approached.

It has become clear to us from our experience in working with schizophrenic patients and their families that the realities of clinical practice are much more complex and demanding than would be first apparent from reading the outcome literature. In Chapters 8 and 9, three areas that may be especially problematic are addressed: the engagement and maintenance of the family in treatment; aggressive and violent behaviour; and the risk of suicide. Although there are no easy ways to resolve these difficult and complex issues, we have suggested ways in which the therapist may try to understand and alleviate these problems.

It should be emphasized that there is a great deal of overlap between these topics; although they appear as discrete categories, they all represent continuous and dynamic processes rather than static, time-limited components. Emphasis is placed on the importance of the patient, relatives, and mental health professionals joining together in a collaborative endeavour to assess the family's individual and collective needs, and to formulate ways of reducing the impact of the illness.

In Chapter 10 we briefly outline two psychosocial approaches which have received considerable attention in recent years: firstly, a psychological method of reduce residual and drug-resistant, positive psychotic symptoms based on the enhancement of coping skills (one author has just completed a controlled evaluation of this method and demonstrated significant reductions in hallucinations and delusions in patients who were not responding further to neuroleptic medication); secondly, the area of the identification of prodromal signs of relapse and their implication for early intervention. Both areas show considerable promise, and could potentially be used in combination with family interventions.

Lastly, in Chapter 11 we briefly address the issue of working within health service organizations, and how to implement a family intervention service.

A comprehensive reference list is provided, as well as suggested further reading. The appendices include a number of assessment instruments that clinicians may find useful; including the Relative Assessment Interview; the Family Questionnaire, the Social Functioning Scale (Birchwood *et al.*, 1990); the Personal Functioning Scale; the Knowledge About Schizophrenia Interview and Scoring Schedule.

Theoretical Perspectives
and Rationales

Chapter 1

Developments in the Understanding and Management of Schizophrenia

As with all innovations, family interventions have emerged from a complex backdrop of different influences. The development of different models of schizophrenia; advances in pharmacological treatments; changes in attitudes to and philosophies of mental health services; the rise of consumerism in mental health; and developments in social psychiatry and clinical psychology have all played their part in determining the context of family interventions.

At this point it is useful to cover some of the background material to schizophrenia. This will be by necessity somewhat brief, but a further reading list is included at the back of the book (page 255).

HISTORY OF THE DIAGNOSIS OF SCHIZOPHRENIA

It appears to be a facet of human nature to try to explain the behaviour of others, especially if it appears abnormal or deviant. The concept of mental illness and the various diagnostic groups it subsumes has been one method of doing this.

Descriptions of abnormal behaviour and psychological disorders go back to antiquity. The medicalization of such disorders developed with great rapidity during the eighteenth and nineteenth centuries with the advance of medical science and the establishment of psychiatry as a branch of medicine. In the late nineteenth century, Emil Kraepelin integrated the work of Morel, Kahlbaum, Hecker, Fink, and others. He described dementia praecox, which developed in early adult life, as characterized by a clinical picture of thought blocking, negativism, impaired judgement, decreased psychological productivity, motor impairment, loss of energy, and affective dysfunction. Kraepelin differentiated dementia praecox from other organic and functional psychoses, its chief characteristic being an inevitable development into a dementing state.

Eugene Bleuler later challenged many of the ideas of Kraepelin, and also changed the name of the disorder to schizophrenia, which literally means, from the Greek, split mind. Bleuler considered the term dementia praecox to be misleading, since the disorder did not always occur in late adolescence or early adulthood, nor did it inevitably always result in a deteriorating course. He thought that cognitive processes, especially looseness of associations, were central to the disorder. Many of his ideas have strong similarities to those now extant in modern cognitive psychology.

The conceptualization of schizophrenia advanced by Bleuler – of a constellation of primary and secondary symptoms which represent a number of disorders with common characteristics – formed the basis of a diagnostic system for schizophrenia. This system was further advanced by German psychiatrists, especially Schneider, who enumerated first- and second-rank symptoms of schizophrenia. The presence of any first-rank symptom was a sufficient criteria in the Schneiderian system for a diagnosis of schizophrenia.

Differences in practice between the various European and North American schools as to what constituted the diagnostic criteria for schizophrenia continued to hamper the study of the disorder until the 1970s. These differences impaired the development of comparative research because different research groups were using differering diagnostic procedures, which compromised the comparability of the findings. This resulted in a difficulty in interpretation of research results, and hence in our knowledge about schizophrenia in general.

To rectify this difficulty, a number of rigorous diagnostic systems were developed over the last two decades. Initially these were used principally for research purposes, although they have had an increasing influence on clinical practice. Well-known examples of these diagnostic systems include the Research Diagnostic Criteria (RDC), and DSM III and DSM III-R, which were developed in the US, and the PSE-CATEGO system, developed in the UK. These systems have narrower, and hence more reliable, criteria for schizophrenia than the diagnostic systems used previously.

Studies carried out in the 1970s, especially in the US, found that the diagnosis of schizophrenia was carelessly applied and grossly over-inclusive. The use of the term 'schizophrenia' is now, hopefully, more reliable, however, it is worth mentioning that a diagnosis produced from one of these systems can on occasions differ from that produced by clinical judgement. This can result in a number of difficulties, especially in the giving of information to relatives.

A further increase in diagnostic rigour has been due to the development of standardized interviewing procedures that can be used to elicit symptoms, for example, the Diagnostic Interview Schedule (DIS); the Structured Clinical Interview for the DSM-III-R (SCIO-R); the Composite International Diagnostic Interview (CIDI); and the Present State Examination (PSE) for the CATEGO system (other relevant methods of assessment of psychopathology are described in Chapter 4). For the purposes of family interventions, these diagnostic and interview systems serve to standardize diagnostic criteria and symptom elicitation. The authors have had considerable experience with the PSE interview, and we have found it excellent for both eliciting symptoms and providing diagnostic information.

The reliability of the diagnosis of schizophrenia to an acceptable level can now be demonstrated. However, this does not necessarily mean it has any validity. Does a diagnosis of schizophrenia actually mean anything? During the 1960s, the anti-psychiatry movement was vociferous in its debate about whether schizophrenia existed or not. This attack came from a number of different sources, and many of the arguments contained certain truths, such as the poor reliability of the diagnosis at that time; the unpleasant consequences of being diagnosed or labelled schizophrenic; and the over-medicalization of both mental health and everyday problems. Many of these difficulties have since been addressed, and many of the criticisms were more properly directed at poor practice and the abuse of the concept of schizophrenia rather than the concept itself. However, the debate about the validity of schizophrenia is still a lively one (Bentall *et al.*, 1988).

The utility of the diagnosis will eventually be determined by its value in clarifying aetiological and therapeutic considerations. Our view is an essentially practical one: since the term is universally used to describe a disorder that is characterized by a reliably identifiable group of symptoms, it has heuristic value. The concept is useful in helping to stimulate debate and research about the disorder and its consequences. Furthermore, it is difficult to abandon both the term and the concept in the absence of any viable alternatives.

CHARACTERISTICS OF SCHIZOPHRENIA

In terms of their experiences, most schizophrenic patients describe sensory disturbances or hallucinations. By far the most common of these are auditory hallucinations, which are experienced by about two-thirds of sufferers. Much less frequent are visual hallucinations, and hallucinations of smell, taste, and touch, which are experienced by about 10–15% of sufferers.

Some schizophrenic patients experience thought disorder, which frequently results in an incapacity to use direct communication, especially language, in an appropriate manner. Delusional ideas are also very common, and these may be of a variety of types, such as, persecutory, delusions of reference, grandeur, and sometimes of control.

The importance of symptoms to the diagnosis of schizophrenia is still the subject of much debate and controversy. The development of rigorous research instruments has greatly increased the reliability and conformity of diagnosis, but opinions still vary on the nature of diagnostically importants symptoms. The experience of hallucinations or delusions *per se* is not generally accepted to be sufficient to receive a diagnosis of schizophrenia. Specific types of hallucinations, delusions, and thought disorder are required to indicate that the diagnosis of schizophrenia is appropriate.

The situation is further complicated by the fact that different illness episodes may be characterized by different types of symptom clusters. Patients may present with symptoms characteristic of schizophrenia on one occasion, and symptoms that are more characteristic of mania or psychotic depression during another. These are the kinds of real-life confusions that lead to diagnostic ambiguities, and which the sufferer and their relatives find so confusing.

Core Symptoms

The symptoms that are generally regarded as core symptoms have been derived from the PSE/CATEGO system, which is widely used in Europe (Wing *et al.*, 1974). They correspond closely with the first-rank symptoms as described by Schneider, and are as follows.

Auditory Hallucinations

1. Voice(s) commenting on the subject's thoughts or actions. The voice(s) speak about the subject and refer to her or him in the third person.
2. Voices talking to each other about the subject, again referring to her or him in the third person.

Delusions of Influence

1. With delusions of control, the subject feels he or she is under the control of some force or power other than him/herself. He or she may feel impulses to say or do things which are not of their own will, such as speaking, moving, writing. This is a basic experience, and the subject may give further delusional elaborations, for example, they are possessed by the Devil.
2. With somatic passivity, an external and alien force has penetrated the subject's mind or body, for example, alien thoughts, X-rays, or radio transmitters implanted inside the subject's teeth.

Thought Disorders

1. In thought insertion, the subject experiences alien thoughts that are recognized as not their own.

2. In thought broadcast, the subject hears his or her thoughts spoken out loud, or believes the thoughts are broadcast so that other people can hear them.

3. With thought block or withdrawal, the subject experiences a sudden, unexpected stopping of their thoughts. This is not due to anxiety or an emotional state. The subject may feel thoughts have been removed from his or her head.

Although these are key diagnostic symptoms in the PSE/CATEGO system, others, such as extensive delusional elaborations, and disruptions to and incoherence of speech and language, may also be present, probably as a result of these basic experiences.

In North America, a greater standardization of diagnostic practice has been achieved through the development of various versions of the Diagnostic and Statistical Manual (DSM) of the American Psychiatric Association, now in the revised version of the third edition (DSM-IIIR). A fourth revision is expected in the near future. The DSM-IIIR criteria for schizophrenia are as follows:

A Presence of characteristic psychotic symptoms in the active phase: either 1., 2., or 3. for at least one week, unless the symptoms are successfully treated:

1. Two of the following:
   (a) delusions;
   (b) prominent hallucinations throughout the day for several days or several times a week for several weeks, each hallucinatory experience not being limited to a few brief moments;
   (c) incoherent or marked loosening of associations;
   (d) catatonic behaviour;
   (e) flat or grossly inappropriate affect.
2. Bizarre delusions, which would be regarded as implausible within the person's culture, e.g., thought broadcast or being controlled by a dead person.
3. Prominent hallucinations, which are not related to mood.

B During the course of the disturbance, functioning in such areas as work, social relations, and self-care is markedly below the highest level achieved before the onset of the disturbance.

C Schizoaffective disorder and mood disorder with psychotic features have been ruled out.

D Continuous signs of the disturbance for at least six months.

The DSM-IIIR also makes a classification on the phase, (e.g., prodromal phase, active phase and residual phase), and the course of the illness, (e.g., subchronic, chronic, chronic with acute exacerbations, in remission).

The DSM-IIIR is now widely used. As can be seen, it is somewhat wider in its definition of schizophrenia than the PSE/Catego system, and includes a six-month duration of the illness as an inclusion criterion.

Negative and Positive Symptoms

The characteristics of schizophrenia which have been described so far – hallucinations, delusions, and thought disorder – are frequently termed positive symptoms or productive symptoms because they are pathological by their presence. A distinction is frequently made between these excesses and what are commonly termed negative symptoms, referring to deficits in functioning, such as flatness of emotion; inattention; lack of motivation and apathy; poor concentration and attention; social withdrawal; restricted levels of speech and communication; decrease in activity level; and an inability to obtain enjoyment from activities. Some workers have suggested a third category of symptoms, which are characterized by cognitive disorganization, such as types of thought disorder, but this three-category system is not as yet widely used.

The negative symptoms of schizophrenia can co-exist with positive symptoms, but they frequently persist in the absence of positive symptoms. They are commonly thought to be difficult to treat, rarely responding well to medication, and some authorities (Crow, 1980a) regard negative symptoms to be characteristic of a more chronic and irreversible syndrome. Negative symptoms are also the cause of considerable social disability and handicap, and are a great source of confusion for relatives, who rarely recognize them as part of the illness. This point is worth emphasizing, since relatives find the emotional and behavioural deficits of schizophrenia very difficult to both understand and cope with. Relatives frequently feel the sufferer is in control and acting on their own volition, hence a lack of activity, conversation, or emotion is attributed to the sufferer rather than to the illness, and becomes a focus of criticism and dissatisfaction.

VULNERABILITY-STRESS MODELS OF SCHIZOPHRENIA

The development of vulnerability-stress models of schizophrenia have been a great advance in both theoretical and practical terms. These ideas have been eloquently advocated by, among others, Zubin and Spring, Nuechterlein and Dawson, and Liberman and Goldstein and their colleagues (Zubin et al., 1977; Liberman, 1982; Nuechterlein et al., 1984; Nuechterlein, 1987; Goldstein, 1990). The vulnerability-stress model has been postulated both as an aetiological model and as an explanation of relapse. We are concerned here more with explanations of relapse or recurring episodes than with aetiology, since one of the main objects of the programme described in this text is to prevent relapse.

In essence, this conceptualization of schizophrenia states that both positive and negative symptoms, and the disabilities and handicaps that arise because of them, are a result of the consequences of environmental stress reacting with an underlying predisposition the individual may have to develop the disorder. Although it is implied that both positive and negative symptoms are incorporated in this explanation, in practice the model usually refers to episodes of positive symptoms, and the mechanisms by which negative symptoms may emerge are less well articulated.

The predisposition to develop schizophrenia is thought to be an enduring vulnerability trait, probably determined by genetic factors. Evidence also suggests that there are dysfunctions in the neurotransmitter systems, probably in the dopaminergic system, and in some cases possibly abnormalities in brain structure. This latter point is the source of some debate at the present time, and is somewhat less well established than the former. For example, the British psychiatrist Tim Crow has put forward the theory that positive symptoms are associated with a dysfunction in the dopamine system, whereas negative symptoms are the result of abnormalities in brain structure (Crow, 1980b). As yet, the evidence for this dichotomy in the disorder is equivocal.

In terms of psychological function, it appears that schizophrenia is associated with a dysfunction or dysfunctions in information processing, which results in an inability to allocate attentional resources and to process environmental stimuli correctly. The exact nature of this dysfunction is unknown, but it appears to render the sufferer vulnerable to stimulus overload.

Considerable evidence suggests that schizophrenia is also associated with a dysfunction in the nervous system's arousal system (Dawson *et al.*, 1984, 1989). Again, it is not clear whether there is a deficit within the arousal system itself, or whether the problem lies in the regulation of the system. The result is that sufferers of schizophrenia frequently show very high levels of physiological arousal, and a tendency to respond dramatically to stimuli in their environment with further increases in arousal. It is postulated that the arousal and information-processing functions are closely related, high levels of arousal being associated with a disruption to information processing and cognitive functions.

It is possible that the disruption to these basic psychological processes results in psychotic symptoms as experienced by the sufferer. A causal link could be proposed between the environment and the levels of stress the sufferer experiences within that environment, through the resulting levels of physiological arousal and information system dysfunction, to the manifestation of schizophrenic symptoms. It should be said that at this point in time the evidence for such a causal chain is tentative, rather than established.

In summary, schizophrenia is the result of a genetically loaded vulnerability that results in dysfunctions within the brain's neurotransmitters, and functionally impairs the information-processing and arousal systems. These psychobiological factors are interactive, with influences resulting from the suffer's environment. The susceptibility to environmental stress means that the nature of the environment is crucial. At present we know more about the effects of environment on relapse once the illness is manifest than about its role in the initial development of the illness.

The possible interaction between an underlying biological vulnerability and environmental stress is represented in Figure 1.1. It represents a threshold model in which the addition of environmental stress and underlying vulnerability may or may not reach a cut-off point. If the

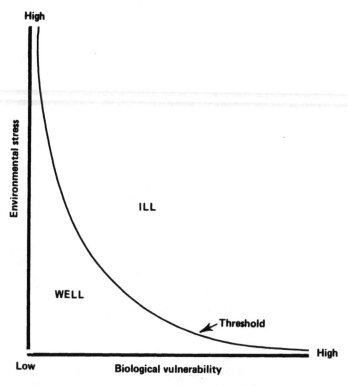

Figure 1.1 Relationship Between Biological Vulnerability and Environmental Stress. (Adapted with permission from Zubin *et al.*, 1983)

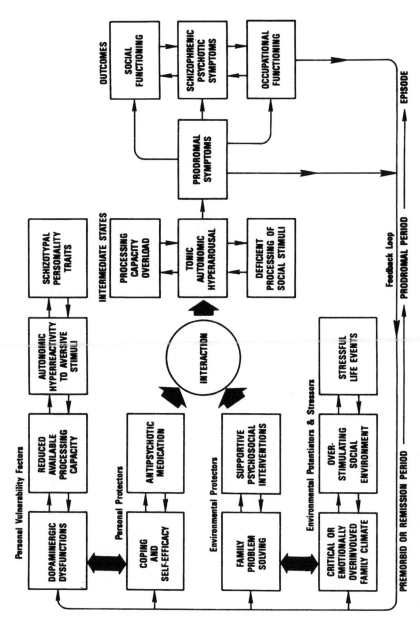

Figure 1.2 A Schematic Articulation of the Vulnerability-Stress Model. (Reprinted with permission from Nuechterlein, 1987)

threshold is reached, then the person becomes ill; if not, they remain well. The degree of vulnerability determines the amount of stress needed to become ill. The illness can only become manifest if vulnerability is present, hence stress alone cannot result in schizophrenia. The more vulnerable the person is, the less stress they need to experience before they reach the well/ill threshold.

This simple model is a useful way of conceptualizing both the initial episode and the precipitation of subsequent relapse. As an explanation of relapse, this heuristic model works quite well, since if a person has already had one episode of schizophrenia, then by definition a vulnerability of some degree must be present. It is also a helpful way to explain to relatives about the episodic nature of schizophrenia, and the varying contributions of genetic/biological and environmental factors. As a complete explanation of schizophrenic episodes, the model is clearly inadequate and too simple. On the one hand, it tells us nothing about the nature of stress or vulnerability nor how to quantify either of these dimensions; and on the other hand, it treats a schizophrenic episode as an all-or-none discrete phenomena, which does not necessarily always reflect clinical observation.

A number of more complex models have been put forward by Keith Nuechterlein and his colleagues (Nuechterlein, 1987; Goldstein, 1990). For example, in Figure 1.2, the essential idea of an interaction between environmental and biological factors is retained, but the various aspects of the model are specified in much greater detail.

The importance of these models is that they emphasize the role of environmental factors, especially social environments, in influencing the course of the illness. Social environments can influence the course of the illness for better or worse, as indicated in Figure 1.2. If social factors are responsible for precipitating relapses, then they can, at least in theory, be identified and modified to reduce the risk of relapse. This supposition has been the driving force behind family interventions.

Supportive and positive social and family environments are thought to be protective factors, while environments that are emotionally charged, involve interaction with hostile or critical people, or are generally over-stimulating are thought to increase the probabilities of relapse. Family interventions aim to promote and facilitate the positive aspects of the social environment. In practice this means identifying the positive and negative consequences of people's behaviour, and attempting to maximize the positive and minimize the negative.

The importance of the vulnerability-stress model to all psychosocial interventions and treatment approaches with schizophrenia cannot be underestimated. Its role with schizophrenia has been compared by the psychologist Graham Turpin to the role of learning theory in the development of behavioural treatments of anxiety and phobias

(Clements *et al.*, 1991). The vulnerability-stress model provides the theoretical drive and direction to clinical practice and research.

TREATMENT

Medication

The conceptualization of schizophrenia as a mental illness, and the predominant involvement of psychiatric medicine in its management, has had implications for treatment. In the 1950s, pharmacological treatments changed quite dramatically with the introduction of neuroleptic drugs. Before this development, medical treatments had had little success in controlling the symptoms of schizophrenia. In many cases management was custodial rather than therapeutic, involving hospitalization – frequently for long periods – in psychiatric institutions.

During the post-war years, a number of factors coincided, resulting in the philosophy of care in the community that is more prevalent today. Firstly, the introduction of neuroleptic medication produced great advances in decreasing the positive symptoms (the experiential symptoms of hallucinations, delusions, and thought disorder) and the disturbed behaviour that was frequently associated with these symptoms. This enabled many sufferers to return to and spend more time in the community. At the same time as this pharmacological advance, there was a general recognition of the detrimental effects of institutionalization, and a public concern about the conditions and practices that existed in some psychiatric hospitals.

Other developments were also important, which would later form the foundations for psychosocial interventions. A number of different strands of research within social psychiatry were beginning to demonstrate the importance of social environments and social factors on the development and course of various mental illnesses and psychological problems. This was especially true of schizophrenia, in which research showed that sufferers were sensitive to the amount of stimulation and stress in their environment: both over-stimulation and under-stimulation could have deleterious effects. Researchers and clinicians were becoming interested in the effects of environments, especially social environments, and how these could influence whether someone remained well or became ill. The possibilities for some kind of therapeutic intervention were clear.

Attitudes within medicine generally were also beginning to change, and a restrictive biomedical model was being challanged (Engel, 1977). Furthermore, models of schizophrenia that posited an interaction between a biological predisposition and environmental stress were becoming more attractive, both to incorporate the increasing quantity of research data, and to suggest new and innovative intervention and treatment methods.

Although neuroleptic medication is still the mainstay of treatment for schizophrenia, its deficits as well as its advantages have become apparent. Many patients experienced unpleasant and unwanted side-effects, some of which were irreversible, and the possible problems of maintaining people on such powerful drugs for long periods were becoming recognized. Furthermore, many patients would discontinue their medication or adhere to treatment regimens in a spasmodic fashon.

Even in drug-compliant patients, follow-up studies suggest that 30–50% would relapse over the first 12 months after discharges, and 40–60% over the first two years (Falloon *et al.*, 1978; Hogarty *et al.*, 1979; Schooler, 1980). Investigations carried out both with patients living in the community and with long-stay patients in psychiatric hospitals showed that even with fairly aggressive pharmacological treatment, up to 50% continued to experience hallucinations and delusions, even if at a reduced and residual level (Silverstein *et al.*, 1978; Curson *et al.*, 1985, 1988). Moreover, although clinical trials have demonstrated that 70% of patients show a clear improvement on neuroleptics, approximately 20% show only minimal improvements, and another 20% appear to remain well on placebo. Furthermore, these results mainly refer to improvements in the positive symptoms, and neuroleptics appear to have little systematic effect on the negative symptoms or deficit states. Neuroleptic medication, although consistently shown to be superior than placebo in double-blind clinical drug trials, does have quite severe and worrying failings as a comprehensive treatment approach.

Community Care

Community care approaches, besides being underpinned by management and treatment issues, have also been supported by political and economic initiatives. Although these have not always been for the most philanthropic of motives, they have produced a climate in which a 'search for alternatives' has been encouraged.

Custodial care in psychiatric institutions gave way to short hospitalizations on acute wards, frequently in general hospitals. However, in many cases this resulted in the 'revolving door' phenomena, in which sufferers experienced a cycle of hospitalization for an acute episode, discharge, followed by relapse and readmission. In addition, chronic long-stay populations within the psychiatric hospitals were frequently maintained by the build up of the 'new long-stay' population.

Because hospital care is expensive and frequently inefficient, new approaches to management within a community setting are being sought. As always, different influences are active, and spectrums of professional opinion exist, from those supporting traditional hospital care to those advocating complete community management. Fears of the relatives that they would shoulder the burden of care in a time of economically depleted community-based service were very real.

Despite all these difficulties and dangers, a radical approach to community care is possible. It is feasible to derive practical management approaches from theoretical conceptualizations of the disorder of schizophrenia. These approaches need to: adopt interactive models and explanations of schizophrenia; adopt a psychosocial perpective as well as a biomedical one; identify and change important environmental influences to the course of the illness; address the needs of the sufferers and their carers, and hence be sensitive to broader outcomes such as indices of the quality of life; and incorporate the sufferer and their families in a collaborative approach to managing the schizophrenic illness and its consequences.

Family intervention programmes are not an alternative to other mental health services. It is not our aim to propose that they are an economically preferable alternative to professional help, or a way of sweetening the bitter pill of the burden of care that families may be encouraged to swallow as part of an ethos of personal responsibility. Rather, family interventions should exist within a sphere of comprehensive mental health services that offer a range of options and resources to meet needs. In promoting family interventions, the aim is to change and improve services, not to offer a do-it-yourself alternative. Family interventions are one of a range of possible constituents of a community service, a community-based service which would differ from traditional hospital-based services.

SUMMARY

Throughout its history, the concept and definition of the schizophrenic disorder has been surrounded by controversy. The development of more reliable diagnostic systems and methods have improved on the rigour of the concept by more strictly delineating the core symptoms that are necessary for a schizophrenic diagnosis. Improvements in establishing the validity of the disorder have progressed less rapidly. The disorder is defined by a group of what has been termed positive symptoms. However, sufferers are also frequently handicapped by what are termed negative symptoms, or gross deficits in functioning. Theoretical explanations were frequently polarized in their explanatory focus, and were usually inadequate to satisfactorally account for the disorder(s) or produce adequate treatment approaches. The development of vulnerability-stress models that incorporated both biological and environmental factors in explaining both the development of schizophrenia and the occurrence of subsequent episodes has been a watershed. Initiatives in treatment approaches have been strongly influenced by explanatory models of schizophrenia and by ideologies of care. The development of broader and multifacetted explanatory models has coincided with moves to provide care within the community setting, complementing the development in broader and more varied services.

Chapter 2

Family Environments

There is a long history of theories that hypothesize an association between the family environment and the development of schizophrenia. Before the development of the vulnerability-stress models and other psychobiological and biobehavioural conceptualizations, there were two unrelated schools of thought about the cause of schizophrenia. The first argued that there was a purely biological explanation, and other factors were at the best trivial; and the second proposed the existence of a purely psychological cause. In terms of the latter model, a number of workers identified the family as an important cause of the illness. Such writers as Bateson, Lidz, Wynne, and Laing described various patterns of family structure, interactions, and communications, which they proposed were responsible for causing schizophrenia (Hirsch et al., 1975). Some writers, such as Laing, suggested that schizophrenia was a family illness.

Although these ideas were influential, there was little if any evidence to substantiate them; most of the speculations resulted from a few clinical observations rather than rigorous scientific investigation. Unfortunately, the unsubstantiated theory that families caused schizophrenia was widely held among professionals. It resulted in considerable harm to the relationship between professionals in the field of mental health and the families of the mentally ill, the ramifications of which are still apparent today. It also caused the relatives of sufferers untold distress: to have a relative suffering from a severe mental illness was bad enough, but to be blamed for causing the illness added to the family's already considerable burden.

These theories of family pathology have not withstood thorough investigation and have now been largely discredited, although their adherents can still be found. It is essential to make clear to the patient, their relatives, and sometimes, unfortunately, to other professionals, that families do not cause schizophrenia, nor does Expressed Emotion research or family interventions imply this.

EXPRESSED EMOTION (EE)

The research on the effects of the family environment on the course of schizophrenia is almost synonymous with the work on EE. The research on EE began in the 1950s when the medical sociologist George Brown and his colleagues at the MRC Social Psychiatry Unit in London became interested in researching the fate of patients who were at that time being discharged from the large psychiatric institutions (Brown, 1985). They found that patients with a diagnosis of schizophrenia faired worse in terms of relapse and rehospitalization rates if they returned to live with their families than if they lived alone or in some other residential setting. This result was somewhat surprising; it might have been thought that returning to live with the family might have provided a supportive environment compared to a large institution, but this did not seem to be the case. Clearly, this was, and still is in view of community-care policies, an important finding.

In a series of studies, Brown and his colleagues investigated this further (Leff *et al.*, 1985). They were interested in the aspects of the home environment that could be responsible for this effect. An interview schedule – the Camberwell Family Interview (CFI) – was developed, which was used to interview the patient's relatives while the patient was in hospital for an acute episode. The interview covered events leading up to the last admission, and questioned the relative about the symptom behaviours of the patient; their attitude and response to the symtoms; and how the illness had affected relationships within the family. Special emphasis was placed on the occurrence of arguments or irritability in the family, and the interview attempted to assess the quality of the relationship between the relative and patient.

The interview was audiotaped, and from this the measure of EE was obtained. In its final version, the rating of EE consisted of five dimensions: critical comments (a frequency count); hostility (a four-point scale, 0–3); marked emotional over-involvement (EOI) (a six-point scale, 0–5); warmth (a six-point scale, 0–5); and positive remarks (a frequency count). In practice, only the first three measures – criticism, hostility, and EOI – are used to rate EE. In early studies, other measures, such as dissatisfaction, were also included, but these were later discarded because they did not appear to predict relapse. Although not of use in determining EE, indications of dissatisfaction can be useful clinically in identifying family needs and areas for change.

EE is a dichotomous measure, and relatives are rated as either high or low depending on their scores on the three principle measures. Relatives who score six or more (seven in the early studies) critical comments or show hostility (one or above), or who show marked over-involvement (usually rated as a score of three or above, but in some studies a score of four or above is used as the cut-off) are rated as high on EE. Only one dimension needs to reach the threshold for the relative to be classified as high (Leff *et al.*, 1985). Some response patterns, however, are more common than others, for example it is common for relatives to be classified as high EE because they are critical, or critical and hostile, or critical and over-involved; less so because they are over-involved only, and rarely because they are hostile only, or hostile and over-involved.

The CFI is usually carried out while the patient is hospitalized for an acute illness episode. After discharge, it is possible to follow up the patient and monitor their progress, comparing the progress of those who return to live with high-EE relatives with those who return to live with low-EE relatives. Significantly more patients who return to live with high-EE relatives relapse over a nine-month follow-up period than do those returning to live with low-EE relatives.

Although the initial studies suggested that behavioural disturbance and previous work history were related to EE and relapse, the general findings from multiple studies have argued that the association of EE and relapse are independent of severity of illness, with the nature of the home environment, as measured by EE, being the best predictor of subsequent relapse when a patient has had at least one previous episode of schizophrenia. However, the debate on the influence of the patient's illness on relatives' responses continues, and it is likely that the relationship between patients' behaviour and relatives' EE levels is complex. It has also been found that high levels of EOI are frequently related to high levels of warmth, but when this is not so, high levels of warmth alone are associated with a good outcome (Brown *et al.*, 1972).

This research was continued by psychologist Christine Vaughn and social psychiatrist Julian Leff (Leff *et al.*, 1985), who further refined the CFI interview and EE measure and carried out a replication study (Vaughn *et al.*, 1976). Their findings supported the original findings of Brown and his colleagues, and also indicated that two other factors were important in predicting relapse. Firstly, the amount of face-to-face contact the patient had with his or her relatives prior to admission: over a typical week, more than 35 hours was classified as high contact, and less than 35 hours as low contact. The second important factor was whether the patient took neuroleptic medication continuously or not: cessation of neuroleptics for one month or more was considered to indicate the patient was not on continuous medication. Patients who lived with high-EE relatives with whom they had high contact and who did not take continuous medication had very high relapse rates (more than 90%) over the post-discharge, nine-month follow-up period. Patients who lived with high-EE relatives but had low contact and took medication continuously over the follow-up period had greatly reduced relapse rates; in fact, equivalent to patients who lived with low-EE relatives.

The two factors of low face-to-face contact and continuous medication appeared to be protective and additive. Furthermore, neither factor appeared to significantly reduce or affect relapse rates in patients living with low-EE relatives, which was originally interpreted as signifying that these patients did not benefit from medication and could probably do without it. However, relapse rates after two years strongly suggested that even in this patient group medication had a prophylactic effect, and those patients not receiving continuous medication were at greater risk of relapse.

Since the mid-1970s, a large number of predictive studies in many different countries and cultures have been carried out investigating the association between EE and schizophrenic relapse. The relapse rates for these studies are shown in Table 2.1 (Kuipers, 1979; Leff *et al.*, 1985;

Table 2.1 Relapse Rates from Prospective Studies on the Outcome of Schizophrenia and Expressed Emotion (EE)

		Percentage Relapse Rates at 9 or 12 months	
		High EE (%)	Low EE (%)
England			
Camberwell	Brown *et al.*, 1962	76	28
	Brown *et al.*, 1972	58	16
	Vaughn and Leff, 1976	48	6
London	MacMillan *et al.*, 1987	68	41
Salford	Tarrier *et al.*, 1988a	48	21
Scotland			
	McCreadie and Phillips, 1988	17	20
Germany			
Hamburg	Kottgen *et al.*, 1984	41	57
Italy			
Milan	Cazullo *et al.*, 1988	63	27
Poland			
	Rostworoska *et al.*, 1987*	60	9
Switzerland			
Geneva	Barrelet *et al.*, 1990	33	0
US			
Anglo-American	Vaughn *et al.*, 1984	56	17
	Moline *et al.*, 1985	91	31
	Nuechterlein *et al.*, 1986	37	0
Mexican-American	Karno *et al.*, 1987	59	26
India			
	Leff *et al.*, 1987	31	9
Australia			
Sydney	Parker *et al.*, 1988	48	60
	Vaughan *et al.*, 1991a	53	25

*Unpublished study

Hooley, 1985; Koenigsberg *et al.*, 1986; Falloon, 1988; Kuipers *et al.*, 1988; Leff, 1989).

It can be seen from the results that the overwhelming finding is that there are higher relapse rates in patients returning to live with high-EE relatives than in those returning to live with low-EE relatives. The majority of such studies show these differences to be statistically significant.

The measure of EE was designed as a research instrument, and there are a number of serious problems in transferring its use to a normal clinical setting. It is important from both the theoretical and practical perspective for the clinician to have an idea of what EE actually represents. There are three lines of evidence that are important in indicating that EE is an index of environmental stress.

Firstly, the psychophysiological studies that have looked at the patient's physiological reactions to face-to-face contact with their relatives (Tarrier *et al.*, 1979; Sturgeon *et al.*, 1984; Tarrier *et al.*, 1988b; Turpin *et al.*, 1988b; Tarrier *et al.*, 1991). These findings are quite complex and somewhat difficult to interpret. To simplify these results, it is suggested that measures of electrodermal activity represent the amount of activity or arousal in the sympathetic nervous system. In the presence of a high-EE relative, the level of arousal is maintained or increased; in the presence of a low-EE relative, the level of arousal decreases fairly quickly. This result is typically found when the patient is acutely ill or when they are tested for the first time. However, follow-up studies suggest that this response is only maintained in patients who live in high contact with high-EE relatives. It is thought that this physiological reaction is in response to the stress of living with a relative who is critical, hostile, or over-involved, which is supported by the fact that changes in the physiological reaction occur if the relative changes from high to low EE over a nine-month period.

Put simply, it appears that living in a stressful environment results in an increasing and accumulating level of physiological arousal, and a propensity to react in such a way to further stressors. The picture is complicated slightly because the probability of heightened reaction to social stressors may be a predisposing factor to increased episodes of the illness, as well as an intermediary stage in the progression towards relapse. Psychophysiological measures may therefore reflect both environmental and biological or genetic factors. Despite the complexity of the findings, these results are compelling evidence for a stress model of EE.

The second important line of evidence is a series of studies that have linked EE levels to actual behaviour of the relative. It has always been assumed that although EE has been rated from an interview with the relative alone, the ratings made from the audiotape of the interview are related to, and directly reflect, the way the relative behaves in the home environment. That is, high-EE relatives must behave differently from low-EE relatives in order to create the stressful environment that is responsible for causing relapse.

This assumption is actually quite difficult to support. Observing relatives and patients interacting in their homes in real-life situations poses immense methodological problems, which would be difficult to overcome. The alternative is to bring the patient and his or her family into the laboratory and observe their methods of interaction and communication while performing some type of task. Although this is somewhat artificial, it has been reasoned that such family interaction patterns are sufficiently stable to occur even in the contrived environment of the laboratory. These studies have found, not surprisingly, that relatives rated as critical on EE tend to be critical during interactions with the patient, and that relatives rated as over-involved on EE tend to be intrusive during their interactions (Miklowitz *et al.*, 1984; Strachan *et al.*, 1986a, 1986b). It has also been found that high-EE relatives tend to be locked into a series of negative interactions with the patient, whereas low-EE relatives appear to be able to change tack more readily (Hahlweg *et al.*, 1989), suggesting that the patient's behaviour may also be important in determining whether or not the negative interaction escalates. In summary, the studies on relative-patient interaction support the notion that different types of behaviour patterns or styles of interacting distinguish high-EE from low-EE relatives, at least in their interaction with the patient.

The third line of evidence concerns investigations of the relatives' causal attributions about the illness and the patients' behaviour, and how these relate to EE. Recent research by Brewin (1991) and colleagues and by Barrowclough (1991) has suggested that differences between relatives' responses to the patient may be mediated by their beliefs about the illness and symptom behaviours. Using the CFI as a source material, Barrowclough found that high-EE relatives made more attributions about illness-related events than did the low-EE relatives; within the high-EE group, there were differences in the sorts of beliefs that relatives held. The attributions of relatives with marked EOI were similar to the low-EE group, with problems attributed to factors more external to and uncontrollable by the patient. On the other hand, there was an association between high criticism and more attributions internal to the patient, while relatives with hostility ratings also tended to perceive the causes to be controllable by and personal, that is, idiosyncratic, to the schizophrenia sufferer. Barrowclough proposes that high-EE relatives perceive the illness events to have more negative consequences than do the low-EE group; hence they are more active in their attempts to understand and control or master the problems. In these respects, high EE represents a unitary concept, although the kinds of beliefs and controlling responses are binary.

Two broad strategies can be distinguished. On the one hand, coercive attempts to restore behaviour (criticism or hostility, mediated by beliefs of controllable and internal attributions); and on the other hand, intrusive attempts to limit negative consequences, by buffering the patient or doing things for them (EOI mediated by beliefs of external and controllable attributions).

Hooley (1985) and Greenley (1986) have previously discussed the concept of control in the understanding of EE responses. Although more research is needed to test the attributional model, the preliminary work on attributions has provided some supporting evidence. Moreover, its conceptualization of high-EE relatives as people who are trying to make sense of the patient's disturbed behaviour places their responses in a functional context; and the focus on illness perceptions has considerable inplications for intervening with families.

One or two other findings concerning EE are worth mentioning at this point. An early study carried out by George Brown and his colleagues, published in 1972, reported that about one-third of relatives rated as high EE during the admission of the patient to hospital were rated as low EE when they were reassessed after the patient was discharged and in remission. Other studies, notably the Hamburg and Salford Studies, report similar findings (Dulz *et al.*, 1986; Tarrier *et al.*, 1988a).

These results can and have been interpreted to signify that EE is an unstable, and hence unreliable, measure. Another possible interpretation is that EE is only predictive of relapse when it is measured during a critical incident, such as hospital admission or an acute episode. Presumably the occurrence of such a crisis is necessary to evoke the important emotional expression from the relative during their interview. In support of this explanation are the findings from the one published study that assessed relatives' EE while the patient was in remission in the community, and which did not predict subsequent relapse.

More recently, the work of Michael Goldstein and his colleagues in California (Goldstein *et al.*, 1989) have suggested a third and intriguing possibility. They suggest that relatives may be classified into three broad categories: those rated as high-EE during admission and remission (high-high); those rated as high at admission and low in remission (high-low); and those rated low EE. They provide evidence that high-high EE relatives show more negative behaviour when they interact with the patient and evoke more negative behaviour in return than do relatives in the other two groups. There have not yet been any published studies that report differential relapse rates between these three groups, but some of the intervention studies, which will be reviewed later, demonstrate that lower relapse rates are apparent in patients who live with relatives who change from high to low EE during the intervention. Certainly, from the standpoint of the model being proposed, patients who live in households in which negative behaviour and emotions are persistent and stable over

time are more likely to be at risk of relapse due to increases in physiological arousal associated with the experiencing of stressful interactions.

The other important finding suggested by recent research is that high-
EE relatives who are rated as being hostile may be different, or have a
different effect, than other high-EE relatives (Tarrier, 1991a). This has
been indicated by a number of findings. Firstly, that patients who live
with high-EE-hostile relatives have significantly lower levels of social
functioning than those who live with other high-EE and low-EE relatives
(Barrowclough *et al.*, 1990). Although it is not possible to say whether
living with a hostile relative causes low social functioning or vice versa it
is unlikely that a relative who is rejecting and hostile will encourage and
facilitate improvements in the patient's functioning. The second piece of
evidence to suggest that hostile relatives are different is the report of the
two-year follow-up results from a predictive EE study carried out in India
(Leff *et al.*, 1990a). The 12-month follow-up results indicated that higher
relapse rates were associated with living with a high-EE relative (Table
2.1), but at two years this significant relationship was no longer apparent.
Relapse at two years was significantly associated with the ratings of
hostility during the initial admission.

These studies are interesting because they suggest there is more
variance within high-EE relatives than was previously apparent, which
may explain some of the differences in relapse rates from the different
studies.

One more finding concerning EE which may be of interest, especially
in helping to explain the more benign course of schizophrenia in developing countries, is the frequency distribution of high-EE households in the
various studies. There is a trend for less urbanized and less Westernized
populations in developing countries to have a much lower percentage of
high-EE households than the more urban communities in the Western
world (Tarrier *et al.*, 1990a). This is also true of samples within the same
countries, such as Hispanic compared to Anglo-American populations
within the US. One explanation is that less Westernized, more traditional
cultures may be more tolerant of the patient's illness and behaviour than
their more 'developed' counterparts.

In summary, the EE rating of the relative to which the schizophrenic
patient returns to live with after discharge following an acute illness
episode appears to be an important influence on whether the patient
remains well or relapses. EE probably reflects a complex network of
factors, which may have arisen for a number of different reasons. The
final result is to create a stressful environment that causes physiological
changes in the patient. Sustained levels of heightened physiological
arousal results in the return of positive psychotic symptoms and relapse.
The exact mechanisms by which increased arousal influences or produces
the disturbances of perception, attention and thinking that are manifest

as symptoms is not known. Reference to Figure 1.2 in Chapter 1 suggests that relapse is preceded by intermediatary states of hyper-arousal and overload of information-processing capacity, which leads into a prodromal stage. During this prodromal stage, symptoms begin to emerge and intensify until a full-blown relapse occurs. This description does not bring us any closer to knowing how these processes actually occur, but such conceptualizations help to guide our thinking about how schizophrenic relapse may come about.

There is no reason to suppose that stress within the family environment is the only source of stress responsible for relapse. Research into life events or life crises has shown that such events as an illness or death in the family; being made redundent or starting a new job; moving house; being involved in an accident; or even something good such as winning a sum of money, appear to precipitate relapse (Brown *et al.*, 1968; Dohrenwend *et al.*, 1987; Day *et al.*, 1987). Such major changes have also been found to be associated with increases in physiological arousal (Tarrier *et al.*, 1979; Nuechterlein *et al.*, 1989). It is also reasonable to suppose that a build-up of stress in other locations or areas of the patient's life – such as at work, study, or in social or leisure activities – would also place the patient at risk.

Although the focus of the intervention described in this book is focused on the family, other factors should also be taken into account, especially since such extrafamilial stress frequently has a knock-on effect and results in intrafamilial stress. The effects of stresses in the environment, both sudden and intense, such as are proposed to occur after a life event, or slower and accumulating, as is suggested to happen as a result of living

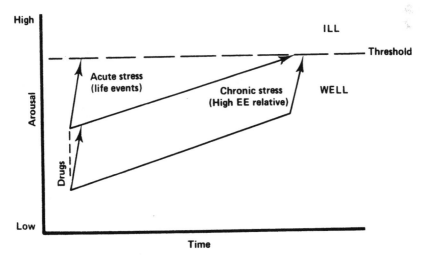

Figure 2.1 Relationship Between Environmental Stress and Arousal.

with a high-EE relative, are represented diagramatically in Figure 2.1. This figure represents the effect of environmental stress, whatever its source, on arousal levels. This again is a threshold model, which proposes a point on the arousal dimension when positive symptoms begin to emerge.

CLINICAL APPLICATION OF EE

The measure of EE and the research it has generated has had a great impact on social psychiatry and mental health. Since the first published studies linking EE to schizophrenic relapse, and especially since the article published by Vaughn *et al.* in 1976, researchers and clinicians have looked for ways to harness the EE measure for everyday clinical usage. The EE measure is problematic in this role, however, and there are strong arguments against its transfer to the clinical setting. These difficulties have been outlined by Smith *et al.* (1990).

Essentially, the use of information provided by the CFI to rate EE is one of classification, i.e., into high or low EE, rather than an enumeration of needs. Furthermore, the implicit assumption is that low-EE relatives are good copers and do not require any assistance or intervention. Unfortunately, such a classification of relatives into high- and low-EE groups can result in a putative, negative label applied to high-EE relatives; and potential restrictions on access to specialist services applied to low-EE relatives. Therefore, as useful as the EE measure may be in a research setting, we do not recommend the rating of relatives' EE levels as the assessment base for a clinical service. This does not mean the information elicited by use of the CFI, nor the EE dimensions themselves are not of use to the clinician; in fact, quite the opposite. We suggest that an interview schedule – the Relatives' Assessment Interview (RAI) – modified from the CFI is a helpful assessment instrument, and that the constituent EE dimensions can be useful in organizing the elicited information. Possible options for the assessment process are outlined in Chapter 4 on assessment; in this section, the ways in which EE concepts and dimensions can be used to generate clinically useful information are described.

EE DIMENSIONS

Criticism, emotional over-involvement, and hostility are the key dimensions that are rated to arrive at a classification of high or low EE. In order to meet reliability standards for replicable research, these dimensions are rigorously delineated, and rules for making the ratings are operationally defined. For example, in order for a critical comment to be rated, a critical tone of voice should be present, or an explicit statement of dissatisfaction must be made. The CFI interview also stipulates that information must be elicited in a standardized way, for example, leading questions asking the relative how they felt about the patient's behaviour are generally avoided.

These two issues – what information is of interest, and how it is obtained – will differ greatly in their focus in the clinical setting compared with the needs of research protocols. For the purposes of assessment that will inform intervention strategies with the relatives, direct questionning of the relative about their reactions to the patient's behaviours will be necessary. A broader information base is sought, since the function of finding out about how the relative has coped with the illness will serve to identify relative and patient needs to be targeted through interventions, rather than to perform a classification. The desired method of eliciting information includes behaviour analysis rather than the CFI/EE rating; however, concepts from the CFI/EE can be relevant in directing an understanding of difficulties in the family context. The following types of information drawn from the concept of EE are potentially of use.

Criticism and Dissatisfaction

In the context of needs identification, the strict distinction between criticism and an expression of dissatisfaction, which is maintained in the rating of EE, is unnecessary. Any topic on which the relative expresses criticism, dissatisfaction, or a desire for change or improvement is of interest. The tone of voice may indicate the degree of dissatisfaction, as it would in any clinical interview, but it is no longer an inclusion criterion. The interviewer should facilitate the respondent to specify exactly what the patient does or does not do, why this is causing concern, and what the consequences are to the family members.

Hostility

Hostile comments are those that negatively evaluate the patient as a person, rather than criticisms of specific things they do or fail to do; they are directed against the person rather than the behaviour. They can be either generalizations from a specific criticism, such as, 'She doesn't do the washing up properly; in fact, she's no good at anything.'; or hostility may be indicated by a rejecting comment, such as expressions of dislike or not wanting the patient back, for example, 'If the hospital sends him home, I'm leaving. I don't want to be with him.' Hostility can be thought of as a more severe and pervasive negative attitude about the patient than just dissatisfactions with specific aspects of behaviour.

Emotional Over-Involvement (EOI)

In the rating of EE, the dimension of EOI is probably the most complex since it involves examples of a number of different behaviours of the relative from which a global rating is derived. Such behaviours can include both the relative's self-report of the way they act, and also the way they behave during the interview itself. EOI therefore rationalizes on to one dimension a heterogeneous collection of different behaviours. In clinical practice we are interested in these different behaviours for their own sake – in terms of what consequences they have for the relative's and patient's well-being, rather than in using them to make a global judgement. Behaviours included in the EOI categorization are detailed below.

Exaggerated Emotional Response

This includes examples of the relative being excessively anxious or worried about the patient or his/her welfare, for example, statements such as, 'I worry about her all the time. I just can't get her out of my mind.' 'I don't know what to do, I've been so upset by her illness.' 'I've been so depressed since he got poorly, I just can't cope.' Also included are over-concern or excessive over-identification with the patient, so that the relative's reactions are closely linked to the patients, for example, 'When he feels down, so do I.' 'Her problems affected me so badly, I had to see the doctor myself.' 'Every time she gets ill, I get taken bad too.'

Self-Sacrifice and Over-Indulgent Behaviour

This includes examples of behaviour where the relative has sacrificed their needs to look after or care for the patient. Examples of this would be the patient's husband saying, 'I gave up my own job so I could look after her (his wife).' Or a mother saying, 'We [the parents] haven't been out [socially] since he [the son] got ill.' Or a mother saying, 'I had to give up everything – family and friends, everything – to look after him [her son]. I can't leave him alone because I worry to leave him. We never see anyone or go anywhere. It's just the two of us now.'

Evidence of the respondent spoiling the patient or being over-indulgent would also indicate self-sacrifice, as demonstrated in such statements as, 'We [the parents] tend to let her [the daughter] do what she wants, otherwise she gets upset, and what with her being ill we like to try and compensate in other ways . . . sort of make it up to her.' Or, 'I [the mother] take all his [her son] meals up to him in bed, but he still doesn't get up.' And from the same mother, 'Because he's been so unwell, I like to do everything I can for him.'

Further evidence of this type of attitude would be if the relative regularly puts the needs of the patient before their own. For example, a mother saying, 'I'd leave him [her husband] if it came to it, so I could look after John [her son].' Or a father saying about his son, 'We [the parents] had to spend all our savings to pay his debts.' Examples of the relative devoting their life to the patient, or their care taking up the whole life of the relative, especially if there is evidence that this is unnecessary, would also be included in this category.

Extreme Over-Protectiveness

Evidence here would be of the relative treating the patient in an age-inappropriate manner, or not allowing the patient autonomy or independence. For example, the father of a man in his 30s, who had just recovered from his first episode, opening his son's letters because he blamed the son's girlfriend for the illness and did not want his son to have further contact with her. Other examples include when the patient is not allowed to manage their own finances, or take responsibility for their own medication; or when the relative will not let the patient go out alone, or in the evenings, or with friends because of what might happen. Or evidence suggesting the relative is being intrusive or interfering in the patient's affairs, even with the best of motives. An example of this is a mother writing to the personnel officer of a firm with whom her son was applying for a job, asking that he be given a 'job without much stress as he had schizophrenia.'

Emotional Display During the Interview

Evidence during the interview of an emotional reaction from the respondent may manifest as overt distress, such as crying or anger; excessive concern; being melodramatic; or in the speech or non-verbal expression.

Emotional Distress

This consists of reports by the relative of emotional reactance or negative consequences to the relative's health because of the patient's illness. These would include statements about their emotional reactions, such as, 'I just cry all the time.' 'I just get so upset when I think about Michael [the patient]. I just can't do anything, it makes me so sad to think about him and his life being in ruins.' 'It [the patient's illness] gets me right down.'

Further indications of distress would include examples of the relative having to seek help or having suffered ill-health because of the patient's illness: 'It was so bad that I had to see a psychiatrist myself.' 'I just couldn't cope with it all . . . I felt so ill myself I just had to go to bed, I couldn't be doing with it all. I felt terrible, so ill.' Or a husband saying that he had to receive treatment for his ulcer, or a mother saying she had to get tablets from her doctor because of her 'upset nerves'.

Extreme Preoccupation With the Patient's Illness

Evidence that the respondent is extremely preoccupied with the patient's illness is suggested when they are unable to talk about other subjects, or they describe illness events in excessive and minute detail.

General

A general pointer indicating that the relative may rate on EOI is the lack of evidence that the relative is displaying 'non-EOI' behaviours, such as encouraging independence and autonomy or allowing the patient to develope their own interests.

Warmth and Positive Remarks

Warmth and positive remarks are traditionally rated from the CFI but are not used in the classification of EE because there is no empirical evidence that these two dimensions predict relapse. For our purposes of collecting clinically relevant information, however, the expression of positive feelings for the patient, and the identification of the patient's qualities and abilities are extremely important in planning an intervention.

Warmth includes statements of sympathy; concern and empathy for the patient; concern for the well-being of the patient as a person; and indications that the respondent enjoys the patient's company and doing things together. A warm tone of voice when talking about the patient is indicative of a positive attitude. Regarding positive remarks, statements specifying the patient's abilities, skills, and positive attributes would be relevant.

CONCLUSIONS

Although it has been emphasized that there are aspects of the relationships between schizophrenic relapse, patient factors, and the behaviour of relatives that are poorly understood, it is worthwhile summarizing these points again since it is important that practioners do not adopt the view that high EE is synonomous with problem families.

Although there is a well-established relationship between EE status and patient relapse, high-EE relatives are a heterogenous group, representing a range of problems, coping styles, and interaction patterns, as well as unique strengths and assets. There are no 'cookbook' answers to the most important targets for behaviour change in relatives, and packages of techniques are premature and inappropriate. Additionally, a cause-and-effect model of EE and schizophrenic relapse is probably over-simplistic, and it would be unfortunate if therapists adopted such a viewpoint. Illness factors – chronicity and severity of symptoms, including behavioural disturbances – may well contribute to the development of problems in families and in difficulties in managing behaviour, and they need to be taken into account when planning interventions. It is also misleading to conceptualize all low-EE relatives as calm, effective copers, who facilitate rehabilitation and reduce the risk of relapses by creating a stress-free domestic atmosphere. Given the severe and pervasive consequences of the illness, one should not assume that any relative of a schizophrenic patient is without difficulties; and it has been suggested that a lack of marked criticism or over-involvement may sometimes be a function of burn-out, with the distancing of the relative from the patient's problems (Vaughn, 1986), or that relapse reduction in low-EE homes may be at the cost of reduced social functioning (Smith *et al.*, 1987). Additionally, it has been suggested that low-EE relatives may develop high-EE behaviours if the patient deteriorates.

These considerations indicate that training in EE assessments is not a necessary prerequisite for working with the families, and a needs-led rather than EE-reduction approach is more appropriate for clinical practice. There should be multiple measures of treatment efficacy, and focusing on relapse prevention may obscure the needs of individual families. However, some understanding of the EE measure is helpful in providing a framework for evaluating coping strategies and in pointing to areas of possible need. The Salford Family Intervention Study adopted an approach whereby the individual needs of family members were assessed, while knowledge about EE informed the therapists' framework for setting priorities for behaviour change. The guidelines set out in later chapters are derived from the Study's intervention format, and apply an understanding of EE to clinical practice.

Chapter 3

Family Intervention Studies

The research done on EE has stimulated a number of family intervention studies. Although these studies differ in detail, they are all based on the premise that if living with a high-EE relative, there is an increased probability of schizophrenic relapse in patients who have had at least one previous illness episode. The studies tested the hypothesis that interventions with the families would reduce this risk factor, resulting in decreased relapse rates. Such intervention trials have all been remarkably effective, except for the Hamburg and Sydney Studies. The relapse rates for the intervention and control groups are shown in Table 3.1. Each of the studies is described briefly below (Barrowclough *et al.*, 1984; Koenigsberg *et al.*, 1986; Kuipers *et al.*, 1988; Tarrier *et al.*, 1990b).

INTERVENTION STUDIES

The First Camberwell Study

Julian Leff and his colleagues in London recruited 24 families in which the patient had high contact with a high-EE relative (Leff *et al.*, 1982; 1985). Families were randomly allocated to an experimental psychosocial intervention in addition to routine care by NHS psychiatric services; a control group received routine care only. The experimental group received an educational programme for relatives about schizophrenia, attended a relatives' group, and received individual family therapy as well as routine NHS psychiatric care. The aim of the intervention was to reduce the EE level of the relative from high to low, and/or to reduce the amount of face-to-face contact the patient had with their relative.

Assessment of relapse after nine months showed a significant decrease in the experimental treatment (8%) compared to the control treatment (50%). Analysis of the relatives' EE and contact time after nine months found that at least one of the above aims had been achieved in 75% of the families in the experimental group. Furthermore, there were no relapses in the families in which these goals had been achieved. Families in both the experimental and control groups received only NHS routine care

Table 3.1   Family Intervention Studies: Relapse Rates for High-EE Households

	Relapse Rates in Percentages	
Study	*9 or 12 months*	*24 months*
Camberwell Study 1		
(Leff *et al.*, 1982; 1985)		
Family Intervention	8	20
Routine Treatment	50	78
Camberwell Study 2		
(Leff *et al.*, 1989; 1990b)		
Family Therapy	8	33
Relatives Groups	17	36
California-USC Study		
(Falloon *et al.*, 1982; 1985)		
Family Intervention	6	17
Individual Intervention	44	83
Hamburg Study		
(Kottgen *et al.*, 1984)		
Group Psychodynamic Intervention	33	
Control Group	43	
Pittsburgh Study		
(Hogarty *et al.*, 1986; 1987)		
Family Intervention	23 (19)	(32)
Social Skills Training	30 (20)	(42)
Combined FI and SST	9 (0)	(25)
Control Group	41	66
Salford Study		
(Tarrier *et al.*, 1988a; 1989)		
Family Intervention	12 (5)	33 (24)
Education Programme	43	57
Routine Treatment	53	60
Sydney Study		
(Vaughan *et al.*, 1990b)		
Relatives' Counselling	41	
Control Group	65	

(Percentages in parentheses represent 'treatment takers' only, and exclude those who did not complete the intervention programme.)

between nine months and two years. At the two-year follow up, there was still a significant benefit of the experimental intervention (20%) compared to the control group (78%) in terms of relapse. However, two patients in the experimental group committed suicide. If these two suicides are added to the relapses, there were 40% treatment failures in the experimental group at two years.

The Second Camberwell Study

In a subsequent study, Leff and his colleagues attempted to evaluate the different components of their intervention package (Leff *et al.*, 1989; 1990b). Twenty-four families in which the patient was in high contact with a high-EE relative were randomly allocated to receive either relatives' groups or individual family therapy. All families received an educational package, and all patients were on maintenance medication, in addition to receiving routine psychiatric care. However, relatives from only six of the twelve families allocated to the relatives' groups attended even one group session.

At nine months, the relapse rates for the family intervention limb were lower (8%), but not significantly different from those who attended the relatives' groups (17%). The relapse rate in the patients whose relatives did not comply with the relatives' groups was high, with three patients relapsing.

Low subject numbers make this study difficult to interpret. The authors have recently reported the two-year follow-up data for this second study: there appears little difference between the relapse rates for family therapy (33%) and the relatives' groups (36%). The authors state that the economic advantages of running relatives' groups in terms of larger case-load must be balanced with the high non-compliance rate and the poor outcome for those who do not attend, of whom 60% relapsed over two years.

When the data from the first and second Camberwell trials were combined, it was found that relapse rates in patients whose relatives show a decrease in either EE and/or contact time with the patient had very low relapse rates (5%) over nine months' follow-up.

The California-USC Study

A study carried out in California by the behaviourally oriented psychiatrist Ian Falloon and his colleagues (Falloon *et al.*, 1982; 1984; 1985) recruited 36 patients and their families, who were identified as 'high-tension'. Thirty-three of these patients lived with high-EE relatives. The families were randomly allocated to receive either an experimental behavioural family therapy group, or an individual supportive psychotherapy control group. The experimental group received an educational pro- gramme, communication, and problem-solving training. During the initial nine months of treatment, each group received 25 therapy sessions, the family management group receiving sessions in their homes. The indi- vidual therapy group also received family counselling and support, but only in response to a crisis. Between 9–24 months, sessions occurred once a month.

In terms of relapse, the experimental group had significantly lower relapse rates (6%) at nine months compared to the control group (44%). The experimental group had significantly more patients in remission than the control group; 44% experienced florid symptoms in the former compared to 77.7% in the latter group; and the experimental group had significantly greater community tenure over the nine-month follow-up period. After two years, the significant benefit in terms of relapse rates between the family management (17%) and the individual treatment group (83%) had been maintained.

The Hamburg Study

In a study carried out in West Germany by Kottgen and Hand and their colleagues (Kottgen *et al.*, 1984; Dulz *et al.*, 1986), young first- or second-episode patients with high-EE relatives were allocated to received group psychotherapy or no treatment. Family therapy was given 'indirectly', as patients and their relatives received the group therapy seperately. A low-EE, no-treatment control group was also included.

Relapse rates for the high-EE treatment group (36%) were lower, but not significantly different from the high-EE control group (54%). This study differed from the others in that a group analytic orientation to treatment was adopted. It has been suggested by Strachan (1986) that the analytic nature of the treatment may have been stressful in itself and resulted in high relapse rates. This study is also unusual in that patients returning to high-EE families show lower relapse rates (an aggregate rate of 41%) compared to those returning to low-EE families (57%).

The Pittsburgh Study

Hogarty and his colleagues (Hogarty *et al.*, 1986; 1987; 1991) carried out an ambitious study in which 103 patients and their high-EE families were allocated to one of four groups. Hogarty had already carried out two large studies in the 1970s examining the efficacy of social case-work which did not show any particular benefit from these interventions, although it was not clear from the published reports of what the interventions consisted, although presumably it was some type of supportive psychotherapy.

In this newer study, the subjects – all of whom lived in high-EE households – were allocated to a control group, social skills training for the patient, psychoeducation and family management, and a combination of social skills training and family management. The control group received medication in a supportive environment. Patients who received social skills training sessions received these on a weekly basis for the first year, and then biweekly or monthly. Skills training was initially aimed at family interactions, but later also focused on outside activities. The family management group initially received weekly sessions during the acute phase, then biweekly 'for several months', and then monthly. The intervention aimed to reduce family stress, increase family tolerance, and re-integrate the patient into the outside world. The combined group received both treatments, and hence had more therapist contact.

After 12 months, the relapse rates were as follows: control group (41%); social skills training alone (20%); family management alone (19%); combined family management and social skills (0%). However, these relapse rates include 'treatment takers' only; if drop-outs or 'partial takers' are included, the relapse rates are as follows: social skills training alone (30%); family management alone (23%); combined treatment (9%).

Follow-up assessments of the relatives' EE demonstrated that: no relapses had occurred in households that changed from high EE to low EE; households that remained high EE at 12 months had elevated relapse rates (42% in the control group, 33% in the family management group, and 29% in the social skills group); only the combined treatment protected households that remained high EE against relapse. Furthermore, it was found that EOI tended to dissappear over follow up; 31% of relatives were assessed as high EE on EOI at admission, but only 6% at 12 months, and it did not appear to contribute to relapse. This is in contrast with the results of Leff and his colleagues, who reported that EOI was difficult to change. Criticism and hostility together were found to be most often associated with relapse: 56% of patients who relapsed had relatives rated as both critical and hostile, compared to 21% of survivors. This result adds further support to the notion that hostile relatives may be different to non-hostile, high-EE relatives.

After two years, the relapse rates were as follows: control group (66%); social skills alone (42%); family management alone (32%); and combined treatments (25%). The authors concluded that relapse had been delayed by the intervention over the first year, rather than having been prevented.

The Salford Study

Tarrier, Barrowclough, and their colleagues (Tarrier *et al.*, 1988a; 1989) recruited 92 patients and their families while the patient was hospitalized. Nine families (10%) refused to complete the assessment and were excluded from the study. Sixty-four (77%) patients came from high-EE households and were designated high risk. 19 patients lived with low-EE families and were designated low risk.

Essentially, a dismantling design was employed. The relatives were viewed as rehabilitative agents, and the intervention was designed to teach them the skills to manage the patient in the home by reducing stress in the environment. The complete intervention included a brief educational programme, which informed the relatives about schizophrenia and gave general advice on how to manage the patient in the home. Since many relatives reported they were highly stressed and appeared to cope poorly with stress, the second part of the intervention consisted of stress management, in which the relatives were taught to identify and modify stresses within the family. The last part of the intervention consisted of goal planning, during which the family's needs were identified and goals formulated to meet those needs.

Two levels of intervention were used. The first – the enactive – included role-playing, behavioural rehearsal, guided practice, self-monitoring, and other participatory methods. A stress-innoculation programme of one session was also given half-way through the intervention, during which coping strategies to deal with relapse were rehearsed. The second intervention – the symbolic – did not include any participatory methods, but only dicussion and advice, that is it operated at purely a symbolic level. No stress innoculation session was included.

The third intervention group received only the brief educational programme (two sessions), which gave information about schizophrenia and general advice on how to manage it. The last intervention group received routine psychiatric care from the NHS services of Salford Health Authority, although the research team did facilitate contact between the family and the psychiatric services when necessary.

The high-risk group was randomly allocated to one of these four intervention groups. The relapse rates after nine months were as follows: family intervention-enactive (17%); family intervention-symbolic (8%); education-only (43%); and routine care (53%). The low-risk, or low-EE, group were randomly allocated to education-only and routine care, and the relapse rates in these two groups were 22% and 20%, respectively. The family intervention was significantly superior to routine care and the educational programme alone. Giving information and advice to relatives did not significantly improve relapse rates in either the high-risk or low-risk groups. The relapse figures for the family intervention includes those who received a minimum treatment exposure of one intervention session. Of the three relapses in the family intervention groups, two of these had dropped out of treatment.

Examination of the relatives' EE levels at nine months indicated that although changes from high to low EE had occurred in the education and routine treatment groups, it was significantly greater in the family intervention group. Similarly, decreases in criticism and EOI occurred generally, but were of significantly greater magnitude in the family intervention group. Hostility significantly decreased only in the family intervention groups.

Alternative explanations for the group relapse rates – other than the effect of the intervention – were investigated. Firstly, while relapse differences could be explained through medication factors, there were no group differences in medication compliance; months without medication; medication dosage in neuroleptic equivalents; or whether the patient received oral or depot injection (random blood tests and neuroleptic assays were completed with patients on oral medication to confirm self-reported compliance). Hence, differences in medication did not appear to explain the differences in relapse rates. Secondly, to test that the family intervention did not reduce relapse by putting the patient in greater contact with the psychiatric services in general, all outpatient contacts with psychiatrists, social workers, community psychiatric nurses, and day hospital and day-care facilities were monitored and recorded. There were no significant differences between the treatment groups on any of these variables. Lastly, all independent life events experienced by the patients during the intervention period were recorded. It may have been possible that the higher relapse rates in the education-only and routine treatment groups could be explained by a significantly higher frequency of life events experienced by these patients. The opposite proved true, however, with those patients receiving behavioural interventions experiencing significantly more life events. It appears that families receiving interventions may learn to cope with unexpected crises.

At two years the different groups were collapsed into three groups, for which the relapse rates were as follows: high-EE family intervention (33%); high-EE control (59%); and low-EE (33%). Readmission rates were also very much higher in the high-EE control group than the other two groups.

The Sydney Study

In a study carried out by Vaughan and his colleagues in Sydney (Vaughan *et al.*, 1991b), 36 high-EE families of schizophrenic patients were randomly allocated to an intervention and a control group. The parents of patients allocated to the intervention group were offered ten weekly counselling sessions. The patients of these families received only standard after-care, as did the control patients, but were not included in the counselling sessions. The workers focused their intervention solely on the relatives, hence they had no contact with the patients or liaison with the clinical teams responsible for their management. During the counselling sessions, the therapists attempted to form an alliance with the relatives; to increase stability and predictability of family life; decrease guilt and anxiety; and increase self-confidence by providing a sense of mastery through education about schizophrenia. In addition, the therapists tried to increase the relatives' problem-solving and communication skills.

Two patients, one from each group, who had experienced high levels of persistent symptoms from baseline, were excluded from the analysis. Fewer relapses occurred in the intervention group (41%) compared to the control group (65%), but this difference was not significant. Similarly, relapses in patients asymptomatic at discharge were higher, but not significantly so, in the control group (64% compared to 25%). Nine patients in both groups were rehospitalized, and there were four suicides in the control group but none in the experimental group.

THERAPEUTIC EFFECTIVENESS

It is difficult to make direct comparisons between the studies cited since they vary considerably in methodological detail and context. It is possible, however, to make a number of statements concerning the effectiveness of various interventions in relapse prevention.

The overwhelming evidence suggests that relapse rates can be reduced significantly over nine to twelve months by family intervention methods. These benefits are still apparent at two years, although there appears to be a proliferation in relapses during the second year if the intervention is terminated.

This raises the question of 'Which interventions work?' The evidence suggests that general support and crisis intervention is not effective. This is indicated by the failure of both social case-work in the two early studies by Hogarty and co-workers, and the control group in the Falloon Study, which consisted of this type of approach, to have a major effect on relapse rates. The failure of the Hamburg Study to show a treatment effect for their intervention indicates that group analytic psychotherapy is also ineffective. The lack of significant results in the Sydney Study implies that the intervention should focus on the family unit and not just the relatives, and needs to be incorporated into comprehensive mental health services. The overwhelming evidence, principally from the EE-based controlled studies carried out in London (Camberwell) and Salford in the UK, and California and Pittsburgh in the US, indicates that prophylactic, family-focused interventions that aim to reduce stress are effective in reducing relapse.

One apparently contradictory finding from the Pittsburgh Study was that social skills training for the patient alone was equally effective as family management over the first 12 months, although the effectiveness of social skills training showed greater deterioration than family intervention over two years. Since this intervention did not include the family, it would appear to contradict the previous statement on family-focused interventions. However, in this study, social skills training was specifically aimed at interactions within the family, which may explain its effectiveness. In the Salford Study we targeted the social interactions of the patient and relatives if there was an identified need. It is worth noting that in a clinical situation – and these research results support this – individual deficits such as social skills should be targeted for change. Improvements in individual functioning may very well facilitate positive change within the family.

There is also strong evidence to suggest that interventions need to be long-term. Short programmes, such as the education programme in the Salford Study, and relatives' counselling in the Sydney Study, did not reduce relapse rates significantly over routine treatment. The two-year follow-up results from the Camberwell, Pittsburgh, and Salford Studies indicates that 9–12 month interventions delay rather than prevent relapse, at least in some patients. The results of the California-USC Study at two years still showed very dramatic benefits of the family intervention, which may be due to the continued intervention over that period. The length of intervention in many of these studies has been dictated by the constraints of research protocols and research funding. In a clinical situation, where it is important to meet the identified needs of individual families, it is quite probable that many families will require intervention for much longer periods than nine months. Some are likely to need continuing contact over extended periods of time.

Two important points from these conclusions that merit emphasis are: short education or counselling programmes do not affect relapse rates; time-limited family interventions, even of 9–12 months, may delay rather than prevent relapse. The implications of both are that many patients and their families will need long-term, continuing intervention.

THERAPEUTIC MECHANISMS

Having addressed the question, 'Which interventions work?', the question, 'Why do they work?' is immediately raised. This can be answered at two levels: 'What is done?' and 'What effect does it have?'

Evaluation at the first level necessitates a component analysis of the interventions. Common to all the successful interventions is the emphasis on educating the family about schizophrenia. Education itself does not appear to reduce relapse, but it probably is important in engaging the family in treatment and helping them to conceptualize the illness and its problems in a stress-vulnerability framework. Other studies have found that education programmes have the effect of decreasing the relatives' reported levels of burden, distress, and anxiety, although there was no effect on the patients' disturbed behaviour, for example, the education programme of Jo Smith and Max Birchwood in Birmingham (Smith *et al.*, 1987), and these improvements may be short lasting. Interestingly, improvements in burden were not related to the amount of acquired knowledge, suggesting the non-specific benefits of education.

Generally, education programmes have adopted a somewhat simplistic view, assuming the goal to be the acquisition of academic information. This approach is unlikely to result in behaviour change on the part of the relative, nor improvement on the part of the patient. More attention should be paid to the initial beliefs and attitudes of the relative, and how these co-vary with their behaviour. In support of this view, Barrowclough and her colleagues (Barrowclough *et al.*, 1987) produced evidence to show that relatives of the more chronic patients were less receptive to education programmes, and would reject new information given by professionals if it did not fit in with their lay conceptualization of the illness. In all probability, education is a continuing process which imparts various benefits and will continue over the whole length of the intervention.

The workers in the English studies were strongly influenced by the research on EE, and their interventions have explicitly attempted to reduce high-EE characteristics of the relatives. In our own study in Salford we incorporated CFI data into the assessments and targeted problem behaviours from the CFI for change, such as patient's behaviour that received criticism from the relatives, or over-involved behaviour on the part of the relative. Hence, we utilized the information produced by the CFI to drive our clinical intervention.

Our approach is not to assess EE and attempt to change high-EE relatives into low-EE relatives, which is not suitable for a service setting for a number of reasons. Rather, we feel that the CFI, from which EE is rated, elicits a vast amount of information that is potentially important and useful clinically. By the use of this and other information a needs-based intervention can be devised. The various dimensions of the measure, such as areas of criticism, hostility, and various facets of over-involvement can be used to identify needs.

In contrast to the English studies, the American studies appear less directly concerned with the characteristics of EE itself, for example, Falloon and colleagues who focus on general skills and abilities of family members to work within the family unit. The intervention of Hogarty and his colleagues appears to bears some similarities with our own in that the importance of stress management and independence of the patient are emphasized.

There is very strong evidence from the two Camberwell Studies, and also the Pittsburgh and Salford Studies, that reduction in relapse is associated with change in the relatives' EE levels from high to low. Although this may be interpreted to mean that the intervention reduced EE, which in turn was responsible for reduced relapse rates, this causal link is by no means unequivocally demonstrated. It is possible that these interventions directly resulted in clinical improvement in the patient and prevented their relapse, and the changes in the relatives' EE were a consequence of this clinical improvement. We cannot state with absolute confidence that EE is a cause or consequence of the patients' clinical state – in all probability, there is a strong interactive relationship between these two factors.

A more productive approach than the detailed comparison of the different techniques of each intervention is to examine their effects on the patient. All workers in the area have emphasized the importance of stress and stressful home environments. A series of studies have attempted to examine the effects of the relatives' EE levels on the patients' arousal levels (page 21). These psychophysiological studies allow us to produce a tentative explanation of how interventions work.

Stressful environments, whether they be in the family home or elsewhere, result in an accumulating increase in the patient's underlying levels of arousal, and a hyper-reactivity to certain social and environmental stimuli. If this hyper-aroused state does not habituate, then eventually a threshold is reached and symptoms reappear. This is presumably because high arousal disrupts perceptual processes and information-processing capacities. Environments are likely to be stressful when they are complex, unpredictable, ambiguous, and emotionally charged, such as living with a critical, hostile, or over-involved relative. Interventions will be successful if they decrease the complexity, ambiguity, and emotionality, and increase the predictability and clarity of the environment.

Psychophysiological research may have the important function of assessing not only the effect of environmental stress on the patient, but also identifying patients with high levels of vulnerability – possibly biological – to frequent episodes. It is feasible that interventions designed to reduce environmental stress will result in a considerable reduction in relapse risk in some patients, but in others with a greater biological vulnerability, relapse may only be delayed in the short term. These two types of patient may have different needs in terms of psychosocial and pharmacological interventions. However, our knowledge of these important factors is very much in its infancy. Developments in both psychophysiological practical assessment and theory may help to clarify this.

Since not all schizophrenic patients are in close contact with relatives, further investigations are required to examine stressors from other sources, how these affect the course of schizophrenia, and whether interventions can be effective. One such area of interest is in hostel accommodation, and what effects the behaviour of residents and staff has on ambient stress levels.

ASSESSMENT AND OUTCOME MEASURES

Despite all of its benefits, EE research has a number of disadvantages. It has been erroneously interpreted as a measure of family pathology, which could result in the labelling and stigmatizing of relatives. It has concentrated attention on relapse as the single measure of outcome, and hence focused on positive symptoms. Furthermore, there is a danger that because low-EE families have lower relapse rates, they are regarded as not having any problems or intervention needs. Lastly, as a research instrument requiring considerable training and time to use, it has always been difficult to transfer EE to a service setting. Therefore, besides the measurement of EE and the identification of positive-symptom relapse, it is crucial that intervention research develops multiple outcome measures.

Social Functioning

Both the California-USC (Falloon *et al.*, 1984) and the Salford Studies (Barrowclough *et al.*, 1990) systematically measured the patient's level of social functioning. Both studies found that patients in the family-intervention groups showed significant increases compared to control groups. In the second Camberwell Study, Leff and his colleagues reported small but non-significant increases in anecdotal reports on social functioning in patients receiving interventions (Leff *et al.*, 1989).

Improvements in the level of functioning are important for a number of reasons: lack of activities and low levels of social interaction both inside and outside the family are a frequent source of criticism of the relatives, therefore, improving social functioning should decrease these criticisms and may produce a positive attitude in the relative; increases in levels of functioning should be related to increased quality of life for the patient, since these improvements will increase the options open to them; poor social functioning is likely to bring about negative evaluations from the public and community in general, and improvements will have a social value for that particular patient and sufferers in general.

The importance of improved social functioning has largely been ignored by researchers. While the clinician should not underestimate its importance as an intervention goal, it should be realized that improved social functioning in the patient may expose him to increased levels of stress as a result of doing more. Intervention goals of preventing relapse and increasing social functioning may conflict, which goal receives priority will depend on the details of the individual case, and the individual patient's decision on the risks. There is an argument, however, that improvements in social functioning and quality of life outweigh the risk of relapse.

Relatives' Burden

There is evidence to suggest that relatives carry a considerable burden in caring for the mentally ill. Controlled trials of community care versus traditional care carried out in the US (Test *et al.*, 1980) and Australia (Reynolds *et al.*, 1984) have not shown that community-based care either increases or decreases family burden compared to traditional care. There is considerable concern, however, that increasing moves to implement community care will result in an increased burden on the family. It is therefore important that family interventions, which place the relatives in an important role as the primary rehabilitative agents, do not in doing so increase the burden on the family.

In the California Study, Falloon and his colleagues have attempted to evaluate this issue (Falloon *et al.*, 1985) by explicitly stating that their goal was to maximize the quality of community life for patients and their care-givers. They found decreases in relatives' subjective burden, social and clinical morbidity, and family coping behaviour for families receiving family intervention. These improvements were explained by the authors as due to decreases in positive symptoms and disruptive behaviour. There is also evidence that perceived family burden was reduced by short education programmes.

Subjective burden of care does not appear to be increased by family intervention programmes; in fact, what evidence there is suggests that it is actually decreased, but clinicians should be aware of the possible dangers of putting more responsibility onto the family. Even if this is not true objectively, it may be perceived that way and result in the family discontinuing in treatment.

ECONOMIC CONSIDERATIONS

Economic factors are becoming increasingly more important in the planning of health services. It is no longer sufficient for the researcher to demonstrate the clinical efficacy of their intervention, the economic viability must also be proven.

Two of the family-intervention studies have attempted some type of economic analysis. Falloon and his colleagues in California (Cardin *et al.*, 1986) undertook a detailed analysis of all direct and indirect costs to the patients, families, health, welfare, and community agencies associated with their intervention. A cost-benefit analysis of the 12-month data showed the total costs for family management were 19% less than for individually managed patients. A much less ambitious analysis of the Salford Project (Tarrier *et al.*, 1991) was undertaken and only direct costs were analyzed. The treatment of patients who received family intervention showed an overall saving of 37% over the high-EE control groups, and a saving of 27% on mean per-patient costs. In both these studies, reducing inpatient days was a big factor in reducing costs, since the major difference in expense is due to the time the patient spends in hospital. The extra provision of the family intervention in the community or on an outpatient basis appears to be a trivial cost compared to that of hospitalization.

These initial results are encouraging since they suggest that family interventions have an economic as well as clinical benefit. However, they are only over a short period of time, and it is not known whether the economic advantages could be maintained over longer periods, although the follow-up results of both studies at two years suggests the gains may well continue.

CONSUMERS AND CONSUMERISM IN MENTAL HEALTH

Consumer participation in mental health services is becoming an increasingly important issue. It can be approached at a number of levels, from using consumer satisfaction as an outcome measure, to involving users and their families in having an increasingly greater say in determining the nature of mental health services. The latter may prove difficult because it is potentially very threatening to professional mental health workers and their employers. Also, the consumer movement is by no means homogeneous or united, and the opinions of patients as to how services should function may differ greatly from the views of their families.

Surveys generally indicate that patients and their families are frequently dissatisfied with the psychiatric and mental health services. It is therefore especially important to try to evaluate both the patient's and his/her family's satisfaction with the family-intervention programme. It could be too easy to obtain statistically significant but clinically unimportant changes, and also find that both the patients and their families were unhappy about the nature and aims of the programme. Such evaluations of satisfaction are rarely carried out, and when they are the methodology is fairly crude.

Clearly there is an essential need for much greater collaboration between mental health professionals and service consumers. The philosophy of family interventions, at least the behaviourally oriented ones such as the Birmingham and Salford Projects, has been of collaboration with the family. Although this is in line with modern behavioural approaches, it is quite a radical departure from the typical medical and psychiatric expert-led approaches to treatment. Outcome measures based on a consumer approach to mental health have, however, been distinctly lacking from family intervention research; and to our knowledge no one has systematically asked the patient their views on family interventions – an unfortunate and perhaps revealing oversight that reflects how easy it is to devalue a sufferer of mental illness. Hopefully, this will be rectified in future evaluations.

SUMMARY

The available evidence indicates that although families do not cause schizophrenia, the way families and relatives interact with the patient and cope with their illness can be important in determining the course of the illness. People suffering from a schizophrenic illness are particularly sensitive to the influences of their environment, hence the social environment in which patients find themselves can to a varying degree precipitate further relapses, or facilitate the rehabilitative process. Intervention programmes have been successful under certain conditions in: decreasing relapse rates, increasing the patients' level of social functioning, decreasing the relatives' burden of care, and resulting in an economic saving for the mental health services.

Working with families in itself may not necessarily be beneficial. Intervention programmes need to provide information about schizophrenia to all family members; teach methods of decreasing environmental stress; and encourage an enabling process that will increase the level of functioning of the patient and allow the resolution of future problems. A family intervention programme should be integrated with the traditional mental health services to provide continuing care to meet the needs of the individual families, which in some cases will extend over a considerable time period.

Practical Guidelines

Chapter 4

Interventions and the Initial Assessment of Relative and Patient Needs

Previous chapters have established the theoretical perspective and rationale for family interventions, and have detailed the empirical studies that give evidence for their utility. Chapters 4 to 8 provide practical guidelines for practitioners who are working with schizophrenic patients and their relatives.

This chapter discusses some of the logistics of setting up the intervention, considering issues such as the likely duration of the work; the advantages of having a co-therapist; and when and where to see the families. The content and format for obtaining a general picture of the problems and needs of a family are then covered in detail. A comprehensive and detailed assessment of the individual and collective needs of family members is essential for successful intervention with the family. This should be a collaborative exercise whereby the therapists assist the family to express and clarify their difficulties, as well as highlighting their strengths and resources.

ORGANIZATIONAL AND PRACTICAL CONSIDERATIONS

Therapists and Co-Therapists

The term 'therapists' refers to the people who conduct the intervention with the family members. No special significance should be attached to this: as clinical psychologists, it merely reflects the term in most common use in our profession. Other professionals might use labels such as 'worker', 'key worker', 'case manager', or 'clinician'. The term 'patient' refers to the person with a schizophrenic illness. Although 'client' might be the preferred and a more appropriate term, 'patient' presents less confusions since both the relatives and the individuals with schizophrenia are clients of the service.

There are many advantages in having two therapists work with a family. These include the fact that deficits in skills and knowledge in one therapist can be compensated for by the other, and vice versa; the support and opportunity to discuss problems with a team member can be extremely useful; appointments at unsociable hours can be reduced if shared with another worker; and it is often useful for two therapists to conduct parallel sessions with different family members. It will not always be feasible, however, for a service to allocate two workers to one family for an extended time period. In such cases, it is useful to try and enlist a helper to conduct some of the assessments and to 'sound things out' with.

Where there are two co-therapists, it is necessary to work together very closely, especially during the interventions. A useful strategy is to allocate one therapist as key worker for each session, whose role includes organizing the agenda for the session and deciding which therapist will introduce and conduct each item, and what the role of the second therapist will be. This minimizes problems such as family members being unsure who to focus the most attention on, or both therapists talking at once, or two conversations taking place simultaneously between sets of family members and therapists.

Time-Scale of the Interventions

The assessments and interventions described are designed to take place over a nine-month period; nine months was used as a cut-off to assess the intervention's impact on patient relapse in our controlled study, and has no other special significance. Some effective interventions may be shorter and others may necessarily be longer, depending on the needs of the family. It may be helpful to think in a time-scale range of 6–12 months for intensive work, with some continued follow-up for an extended time period.

Initially, appointments are best arranged weekly, and usually after about eight weeks – covering initial assessments, education, stress management, and, where appropriate, some goal-setting – might be reduced to fortnightly, and later to monthly. The early appointments are likely to take more time, with meetings where progress is reviewed being less time-intensive.

Much emphasis in the intervention work is placed on the careful assessment of individual families, since the nature of the interventions stem from the analysis of the difficulties and particular resources of the family. Hence time for assessments needs to be earmarked, and requires about two hours for the initial interviews per family member, plus the additional time for organizing the material collected.

Selection of Families

In an ideal service, it would be desirable to offer intensive help to all families with a schizophrenic member. Constraints in your service, however, will make this impossible. When beginning to work with this client group it may also be helpful to take into consideration who is most likely to benefit.

Most of the published intervention studies commenced working with families at the time the patient was hospitalized for an acute schizophrenic episode. In terms of engaging the family for conducting assessments and embarking on new management strategies, this starting point has many advantages. Often the acute episode will have been marked by behavioural disturbance at home, and relatives will be trying to work out why the illness started or relapse occurred, what will happen in the future, and what they can do about it. Thus the relatives, as well as the patient, usually have acute needs at this point. There is a self-evident rationale for embarking on intensive work with all of the family, and a readiness to try out new strategies directed at ameliorating problems and improving the patient's functioning. Additionally, the relatives are already in contact with the services through hospital visits and interviews, and are receptive to people trying to fully comprehend the nature of the problems presenting at home.

There is some evidence that an intensive input for families of patients experiencing their first episode of schizophrenia may be particularly beneficial (Goldstein *et al.*, 1978), and, given that family members have a short history of coping with and understanding the problems, there are advantages in working with people who are possibly more open to accepting advice. Such advantages, however, do not exclude beginning work with families when the patient has a chronic illness course and currently is not acutely ill, nor is the family at crisis point. It is suggested, however, that engaging families at other times may require more attention to alliance-forming strategies and rationales in order for relatives to change existing coping styles.

In our intervention study, we worked only with patients who were receiving maintenance neuroleptic treatment, usually by attending depot injection clinics, or through visits from community psychiatric nurses. The few patients who were receiving only oral medication attended outpatient appointments for regular medication review. Working with patients who are receiving injections or who are regularly taking medication has many advantages, the most important being that their condition is regularly monitored and stabilized.

This does not exclude patients who receive only intermittent medication and their families from benefiting from psychological interventions. Moreover, in the case of patients who refuse to take medication and whose condition is unstable and problematic, it is likely the relatives will need more help and support, and the patients will be more sensitive to stress in the home environment. However, since the efficacy of the pychosocial interventions has been demonstrated as an adjunct to medication, it would be advisable for those beginning intervention work to commence with patients who are prescribed long-term neuroleptics.

Working With Individual Family Members or the Family Group

The family members who have been involved in intervention work have most frequently been the parents, spouse, partner, or siblings of the patient, but this might also include other relatives or friends who either reside with the patient or have regular contact with them.

Although it is often useful to involve all of the adult family members of the household in the intervention work, in some cases this may not be possible. Some members may not be available for appointments, either through choice or because of other commitments. Establishing the availability of family members at the outset is important. Where key members will be unable to attend all or most of the sessions, therapists need to consider to what extent interventions can be effective; however, families should not be excluded from help purely on the grounds that not everyone can attend all sessions. Often individual members can be helped, and when the behaviour of absent members is assessed to contribute to problems, then relatives can be helped to cope with the consequences or to modify the relatives' responses.

It is useful to see family members individually for initial assessments: individual consultations help to establish rapport between the therapist and individual relatives, and family members have the opportunity to assert their own problems, their particular perspective of the situation, and any interpersonal difficulties within the family situation. However, the interactive nature of many problems in the family context is acknowledged, and will be further assessed as the intervention progresses.

A useful format for the assessment interviews is to first see the family together, including the patient if possible, to discuss with them the purpose of the assessments and to allow general concerns to be aired, followed by arrangements to see relatives individually. Throughout the assessments and interventions, decisions may be required as to whether sessions should be organized for individual relatives or multiple family members, and at which sessions the patient should be included or might benefit from being seen alone. These decisions will include issues concerning how to establish and maintain rapport; address individual needs; respect confidentiality; assess and modify interactions between family members; obtain consistent management strategies, and how best to involve a sometimes disturbed patient member.

Where to See the Family

A flexible approach is required to arranging the time and location of appointments. Issues such as time off work, child-care, transport and proximity, privacy, and the personal preferences of clients dictate whether sessions are conducted at home or in the office, and often after-hours appointments need to be arranged. There are pros and cons to working in the home versus the office. People may feel more relaxed at home, but it is more difficult to structure the session in the less-formal atmosphere of someone's house, where interruptions cannot be controlled.

The location of the session may form part of the intervention. For example, for one elderly carer who lived alone with a very symptomatic and behaviourally disturbed son, coming to the hospital for appointments by herself was the first step in reducing contact with her son and having time for herself; and for one house-bound patient, the hospital appointment was initially the only time he left the house alone.

It is a good idea to visit the home at least once in order to understand any constraints the physical environment has on the family carrying out interventions, or the nature of external stresses operating on the family. For example, crowded homes with few and small rooms pose particular problems for people trying to find time to themselves, and also increase the opportunity for stressful interactions; the TV or stereo on at high volume may be extremely irritating in a house with thin walls; and the idea of taking a walk to reduce feelings of tension may be unhelpful and unwise in a deprived and unsafe inner-city area.

THE GENERAL RATIONALE FOR ASSESSMENT AND INTERVENTION

It is helpful for family members, including the patient, to be first seen together, when the purpose of the subsequent work with the family can be outlined. Some general themes to be covered include acknowledging the problems associated with the experience of mental illness, both for the sufferer and for those in close contact with him or her; and the recognition that because mental illness is different from physical illness – in that difficulties cannot readily be 'seen' by medical staff – in order to help the person and those he/she lives with it is necessary to get personal accounts of how the illness affects them. The proposal can then be introduced that the therapist would like to spend time talking at some length with individual members so that he or she might better understand the family's needs; and that these discussions would inform the therapist as to how he/she might collaborate with the family in addressing some of the issues.

The rationale for the intervention should emphasize that since the patient is living at home or in close contact with the family, the relatives have more contact with the patient than the mental health staff. Hence it is important that the staff ensure they support the efforts of the family if they are to help the patient. In our experience, most relatives and patients readily accept this approach, and most welcome the recognition of their rehabilitative role, and the opportunity to discuss their situation and to voice difficulties.

OBTAINING A GENERAL ASSESSMENT OF NEEDS

The general aim of the initial assessments is to assist the family members in communicating to the therapist difficulties associated with the illness, as well as to highlight the relatives' particular strengths and resources. A summary of these problems and strengths will be the end result of the assessments, and will help to clarify the family situation and to provide an outline of the areas that may be targeted for change during the course of the intervention.

Assessment of the Relatives

Because these areas of potential difficulty will be critical to formulating the intervention components, the following assessment themes should be covered during the initial interview:

1. The relative's understanding about the illness, the symptoms, medication, and so on.
2. Distress in relatives and situations, including thoughts, that trigger distress.
3. Coping strategies used to deal with both positive and negative symptoms, and what effect these have on family members and the patient.
4. The consequences of the illness on the relative, including any restrictions (e.g. social life, occupation) and financial hardship.
5. The relationship with the patient, and the identification of dissatisfactions the relative has about particular aspects of his or her behaviour.
6. Areas of strength, for example, an effective coping strategy, social supports, positive relationship with the patient.

Where there is more than one key relative in the household, the effects of the attitudes and behaviours of the other family members on the assessment themes should be noted. Additionally, current life problems of the relatives should be considered, including health, work, housing, or relationship/marital difficulties, irrespective of whether or not they are associated with the illness. Such problems may well have some bearing on the coping resources of the family members.

EE and the Assessment of the Relatives

While a training in the assessment of EE is not a necessary prerequisite for working with families, the behaviours and attitudes assessed as high EE have been demonstrated to be associated with problematic coping strategies in relatives, and may mediate stress and relapse in patients. We therefore recommend that therapists attempt to take account of evidence of such attitudes and behaviours in their assessments (Chapter 3; Leff *et al.*, 1985). The ways in which criticism and over-involvement may be evident in the initial assessments, and how such factors can be used to inform the assessment themes are briefly described below. As always, the aim of the assessment is to identify areas of need that can be targeted for intervention through changing patient and relative behaviours, rather than to diagnose high EE.

Criticism

A critical comment is an unfavourable comment upon the behaviour or personality of the patient. Criticisms are evident from the content of the remarks relatives make, for example, 'He just sits in the chair all day long, and it really annoys me.'; as well as from the tone of voice, for example, 'He just *sits* in the chair, *all day long*.' The overt expression of annoyance or dislike of patient behaviours, and/or a critical tone of voice is used to separate criticism from dissatisfaction. However, since our concern is to identify behaviours that cause the relative upset, misunderstanding, and coping problems, it is not necessary to discriminate criticism from dissatisfaction.

The tone of the respondent's voice can be a useful index of how much the behaviour bothers the relative, but direct questioning of the extent to which the relative is concerned/upset/annoyed by the behaviour; what he/she thinks is its cause; what effects it has on him/her and other people; and how the family responds, would establish how great the problem is for the family. In this way the information can be used to inform the assessment theme, and may later be targeted for intervention through education, stress management, or patient goal-setting components.

Emotional Over-Involvement (EOI)

The EOI dimension identifies a number of specific behaviours and emotional responses that are viewed as over-concern responses. Unfortunately, the term 'EOI' has negative connotations. In practice, it is often hard to judge what amount of concern on the part of the relative would be normal or usual, given that the relative is living with someone whose behaviour is very disturbed, and whose long-term prognosis is often poor. A more helpful way of looking at the EOI dimension is in terms of the relative's stress responses and coping strategies. The dimension identifies a number of responses to the illness that may be understandable, given the severity of the patient's problems, but which are unhelpful in resolving the problems, and may serve to increase the relative's distress. The responses can be divided into distress responses and coping behaviours.

Distress Responses

The relative's behaviour during the interview may demonstrate that the patient's illness triggers strong emotional reactions. For example, the relative may become obviously upset and tearful, or they may report loss of sleep or interference with their everyday activities through worry and preoccupation with the problems of the illness. Where the relative's preoccupation with the difficulties is extreme, the relative may indicate that their mood is dependent on the patient's condition with statements such as, 'When he suffers, I suffer.', or, 'When she's depressed, I get depressed.' Our main interest here is not in discriminating between realistic and excessive concern on the relative's part; rather we are attempting to assess how the relative's well-being and quality of life have been affected by the illness.

Coping Responses

Within the EOI dimension there are two classes of coping responses that may be unhelpful to the patient and relative.

Self-Sacrificing Behaviours
Here the relative indicates they regularly put their own needs second to the patient's, resulting in some considerable loss to their own quality of life. Examples of such behaviours would be that the relative has given up their own social or leisure activities to be with the patient most of the time; has sacrificed their career or given up work to look after the patient; spends a large amount of time doing things for the patient; or makes large financial sacrifices so they can give the patient money, but are left in need themselves.

Over-Protective and Intrusive Behaviours
These behaviours may or may not be associated with self-sacrifice. The relative treats the patient in a way that is not appropriate to their age on issues of independence and autonomy. Examples would be supervising

the patient doing personal tasks such as washing or shaving to make sure they do them properly; opening their letters; vetting their friends; or otherwise restricting their behaviour.

The responses of self-sacrifice and over-protection may be well intentioned, and used as a means of keeping the patient from harm when the relative feels he or she is unable to function independently, or cannot use good judgement because of their illness. However, from the viewpoints of maintaining or restoring relative and patient well-being, they can have considerable and negative consequences: the patient may be protected from risks and harm, but he or she may become overly dependent on the relative, with a consequent deterioration in social functioning; a parallel situation is that of the patient who is over cared for in an institution. The relative's well-being may also suffer, in so far as their own needs are neglected. Thus, rather than putting value judgements on the relatives' reactions to the illness, they can be assessed in terms of their current or likely longer-term effects on patient and relative well-being. In this way, behaviours associated with EOI can be included under the assessment themes, and priority given to the more problematic aspects during the course of the intervention.

Table 4.1 Content Areas for Relative Assessment Interview (RAI)

---

1. Background information
Who lives in the household? (their age, sex, relationship to patient, employment), any recent changes in.
The household composition?
The contact time of the relative and other household members with the patient.

2. Psychiatric history of the patient
Obtain a chronological account of the history of the illness, beginning 'When did you first notice something different about . . .'s behaviour.'
For all problems or symptoms mentioned, ask about onset, severity, context, reactions, and effects on the relative and other household members.
Note hospital admissions and the reactions of the relative to these.

3. Current problems/symptoms
Has the patient experienced problems with sleep/appetite/bodily complaints/ under or overactivity/slowness/withdrawal/fears-anxiety/worry/depression/self-care/delusions/hallucinations/odd behaviour/finances/drugs or alcohol? The nature, severity, frequency of the problems and relatives reactions and coping responses as well as those of other family members should be ascertained.

4. Relationships between family members
Irritability/tension or quarrelling from or between members of the household (including the patient) should be assessed.

5. General information about the relative
Social, occupational activities and interests of the relative; relationship with the patient and other household members; how relationships and activities and interests have been affected by the illness.

METHODS OF ASSESSMENT

The Interview

The chief method of obtaining information about the family members will be through individual interviews. The Relative Assessment Interview (RAI), (Appendix 1) is based closely on the Camberwell Family Interview (CFI), with some modifications for clinical use. Some of its important content areas are listed in Table 4.1.

Given that in this context the RAI is being used to obtain information to help direct a family intervention, rather than to categorize family members for research purposes, the interviewer may use his or her judgement on the precise nature of the questions used, and the order in which they are asked. Where the practitioner already knows the family well, he/she may feel it is unnecessary to complete some sections, or that further adaptation of the interview is desirable. Such procedures are perfectly acceptable: the aim is to collect information about relatives' needs rather than to complete a standardized procedure.

It is recommended that interviewers have training and experience in reflective listening and paraphrasing, and in cognitive behavioural interviewing (Hawton *et al.*, 1989). Reflection and paraphrasing are important in letting the relative know you have heard what they are saying, and for confirming that you have understood what has been said. They also encourage the relative to communicate with you, and the relative's perception that you are understanding their situation will help to form the alliance that will be important for interventions. Direct questioning and probes are important for pinpointing and analyzing the behaviour of family members, and clarifying the situations in which problems occur. For example:

> Therapist: 'So you get very upset when Alan gets on at Jane for not going out?'
>
> Mother: 'Yes, but it's not that I don't think Jane should go out, it's just that I don't think going on at her helps, and Alan is usually sorry he did it afterwards.'
>
> Therapist: 'Could you give me an example of when this happened recently, when Alan got on at Jane?'

Content Areas of the Interview

Background Information

The interview begins by getting routine details about the composition of the household. It is then useful to establish a timetable of the relative's contact with the patient. From this an idea of the routine of the patient may be formed, for example, identifying patients who spend a lot of time in bed or alone and thus are not seen much by family members; or relatives who spend most of their time attending to the patient's needs; or, alternatively, those who avoid conact with the patient.

Chronological History of the Patient's Illness

It is often appropriate to next establish the chronological history of the patient's illness from the viewpoint of the relative. It is our experience that many relatives have not previously had the opportunity to recount the illness events to an attentive listener, and giving them this opportunity is helpful in establishing rapport before the analysis of current events.

Since it is the relative's viewpoint which is of concern, such questioning should begin with, 'When did . . .'s trouble first begin?', or, 'When did you first notice something different about . . .'s behaviour?'. If relatives are unsure of what the interviewer wants ('Where do you want me to start?'), they should be encouraged to begin wherever they first noticed that the patient had a problem, and be reassured that the interviewer is interested in their impressions, and not the patient's medical record.

There are huge differences in response to this questioning. Some relatives will go back to early childhood and school difficulties, whereas others only perceive troubles or differences in the days before an acute admission to hospital. If there has been a recent acute episode, more detailed questioning should seek to establish its onset and development, with the reactions of the relative.

From the relative's historical account, during this part of the interview one would begin to collect examples of specific situations triggering stress in relatives; how the relative coped with positive symptoms and behavioural disturbances; their feelings and any dissatisfactions about the psychiatric services; and some information on the relative's understanding of the illness, and the reasons for patient relapses.

Irritability

In this section, the interviewer tries to establish whether family members, including the patient and the relative being interviewed, are ever irritable with each other, or have other problems in their relationships, including arguments. To make relatives feel more at ease with this line of questioning, it is a good idea to emphasize that irritability and arguing are normal in families, and particularly in the context of mental illness. For example, when discussing the presence of irritability in the patient, the CFI introduces this with, 'One of the ways in which this kind of trouble affects people is to make them more snappy, or more likely to fly off the handle at things that wouldn't normally worry them . . .'

After establishing any irritability of the patient, examples of how this occurs, and with which family members, should be sought, as well as any examples of arguments or disputes between other family members. The latter might be introduced by suggesting that most people in families disagree or argue from time to time. Issues that cause the relative to get on, or to grumble, at the patient are also probed for. Such lines of questioning should establish: whether the patient is irritable, and if so how the relative and others in the household respond to this; whether there are particular conflicts between family members, and how these are resolved; if the relative or other family members are dissatisfied with aspects of the patient's behaviour, and if so, how he/she deals with these issues.

Current Problems or Symptoms

A time period of the last three months can be used to focus on current problems or symptoms that the relative perceives the patient to be experiencing in the home or community environment. Since interventions will be targeted at current difficulties, it is important to be clear what is *now* happening at home, and one of the functions of the interview is to help the relative to pinpoint current problems. It is useful to anchor the three-month period to some event, for example 'since Easter', or, 'from Christmas onwards'. A checklist of possible symptoms is contained in the RAI, which can be gone through with the relative. Usually, the relative will have identified some of the key problems in earlier sections of the interview, and the interviewer should acknowledge these in order to let the person know they have been listened to. For example:

'You mentioned earlier that Michael had difficulty sleeping. Has this been the case in the last three months, since about Easter?'
or,
'You told me that when John was ill he lashed out at his dad. Have there been other occasions when John has lashed out at, or hurt people in the last few months?'

Some details of the nature, frequency, and context of such difficulties should be established, the relative's behaviour and feelings in response to the problems, the reactions of other family members, and so on. For example:

Mother: 'He gave me a bit of a shove the other week.'
Interviewer: 'Can you tell me more about that? What were you doing at the time?'
Mother: 'I was just washing up, and John came in to make himself a drink of tea. He slopped the milk all over the top of the fridge, and I said, "Can you wipe that mess up?", and he said, "Leave off, mum", and gave me a push. Not hard, just a shove.'

Interviewer: 'What did you do then?'

Mother: 'I just left it, and he went back to his room.'

Interviewer: 'How did you feel about it?'

Mother: 'I was a bit upset. You wonder, should I have said anything? But he's always making a mess in the kitchen.'

Interviewer: 'Have there been any other recent occasions when he's hit or shoved you, or anyone else?'

Mother: 'No. He's not like that. He'd had a bad day that day.'

A more detailed analysis of the behaviours can be made in later stages of the assessment and intervention. The initial interview aims to establish the broad areas of difficulty, and to develop rapport with the relative by facilitating them in giving an overview of events and their reactions to them. This section of questioning is particularly important for establishing areas of patient functioning that are problematic for the relative, as well as something about their understanding of the patient's symptomatology, and how the family members cope with difficulties.

Household Tasks/Money Matters

Questioning what the patient contributes to the running of the household in terms of practical and financial help again probes the relative's feelings about arrangements, and will establish any dissatisfactions they have, or evidence of self-sacrifice or over-protection.

Interests and Social Activities of the Relative

How these have changed during the time the patient has been ill will be important in assessing the needs of the relative, and also the resources that can be used in helping the relative to cope with problems. In extreme cases it may be that the relative has stopped seeing friends and dropped outside interests because of perceived needs and demands of the patient. Consequences of giving up previously enjoyed activities might include feelings of isolation and depressed mood for the relative, and possibly reinforcement of underactivity for the patient. However, there may be friends of the family who are willing to assist in patient-focused goals, such as helping to encourage the patient to go out.

Information on how the relative spends their time and their social contacts will likely be reported in the course of the interview, but specific questioning as to how things have changed since the illness, and what the relative feels about the changes may need to be probed directly. Similarly, how the relative's relationship with other family members has been affected should be elicited, for example, their relationship with their spouse in the case of parental households, as well as changes in the relationship with the patient.

Administration of the Interview

In full, the interview will take an hour to one and a half hours or longer to complete, since it is often the first time the relative has been encouraged to talk at length about their experiences. More than one meeting may be necessary. It is useful to audio-tape the session(s), with the relative's permission, so that its content may be understood and summarized in terms of the themes and issues detailed in earlier sessions. Additionally, the therapist may wish to incorporate some further direct questions about the relative's knowledge about schizophrenia (Chapter 5).

Other Assessments

Other assessments which are useful following from the interview include:

A measure of psychological distress in the relative, for example the General Health Questionnaire (GHQ) (Goldberg, 1972; Goldberg *et al.*, 1988) or the Symptom Rating Test (Kellner *et al.*, 1973). Many relatives are suffering significant psychological problems in terms of depression or anxiety, and the extent of their distress may not be apparent from an interview. Questionnaires such as the GHQ help identify relatives with more severe problems, who may need direct and immediate help before patient-focused plans and interventions are developed.

The Family Questionnaire (FQ) (Appendix 2) (Barrowclough *et al.*, 1987; Tarrier *et al.*, 1987) is a checklist of patient-focused problems. Forty-nine problems are described with one open 'other' category to allow for any idiosyncratic difficulties. The relative is requested to indicate on three five-point scales the frequency with which the behaviours occur; the amount of distress the behaviours cause them; and how well they feel able to cope with the difficulty. The checklist is useful for validating information covered in the interview, and in assessing what the relative perceives are the main problems. It can also be used as a follow-up measure to evaluate progress and outcomes.

CASE EXAMPLE: ORGANIZING ASSESSMENT MATERIAL

Following the interview and the administration of other assessments, it is useful to translate and summarize the themes and issues concerning the relative's situation in terms of their problems, needs, and strengths. An example is given below. The key relatives were the parents of a man in his late 20s.

Background to the Patient and His Family

The patient, Martin, was a 29-year-old man, who at the time of our assessments was hospitalized for an acute schizophrenic episode. He had three previous hospital admissions with a diagnosis of schizophrenia on each occasion, and had been receiving neuroleptic depot injections since his second schizophrenic episode. The time between his hospital admissions had reduced from 10 to 8 and latterly seven months; his first relapse was associated with medication non-compliance, but hospital records indicated that he had complied with injection clinic attendance since his second hospitalization. He was single, and had lived with his parents and had been unemployed since the second episode of illness, although prior to his illness he had lived away from home and had been in continuous employment. He was in full-time education until the age of 21. There were two other siblings, both married, one living locally and the other in the south of England.

Interviews with the Parents

Background Information and Contact Time
The mother, Ann, was employed full time in her profession and worked shifts. She attempted to organize her work hours so as to spend the maximum time at home during the day with Martin. Prior to the recent illness relapse, Martin's normal routine was to get up late morning, spend most of the day in the house, and to go to bed early. Ann felt it important that she organized some activities for Martin, since he seemed to do very little when she wasn't there. She would encourage him to go out with her on her days off for walks, or shopping, or would try to engage him in conversations at home.

The father, Jim, had been unemployed for the past year, having been made redundant from a skilled job he had for 20 years. He had taken on most of the housework and shopping, but said he was often bored at home, and fairly despondent about finding another job. Although Martin was in the house all day, Jim didn't do much with him since he was occupied with housework or doing the garden, while Martin spent most of his time sitting around or watching TV. However, the two got along together, although Jim admitted that he sometimes felt irritated by the fact that Martin didn't offer to do anything in the house, and felt that his son could to more to occupy himself.

Chronological History of the Illness
The mother dated the onset of the problems to a stressful period in Martin's life in his late 20s. At that time, he had been in a relationship

with a woman who had a child from a previous relationship. Ann felt that this woman was overly dependent on Martin, and had exploited his good nature, and that he had worked too hard trying to give her financial and emotional support. Martin began acting strangely about six months after this relationship finished, although she at first attributed his problems to taking marijuana and drinking too much alcohol. When she and her husband began to realize that Martin might need medical help, there had been a difficult two-month period when they had been at a loss as to what to do. During this time Martin had been missing for weeks at a time, and had disposed of most of his possessions.

Eventually, after an episode when he set fire to his flat, the parents called an ambulance and he was admitted to hospital via casualty and emergency services. He seemed to make a good recovery after his first admission, and Ann still then thought that his problems were due to stress and drugs rather than to a mental illness. Martin had gone to live with a friend in the south of England, but had become ill again, was admitted to hospital there, and had been discharged to the parental home. Since then he had received depot injections. Between illness periods he had seemed lethargic and disinterested in life, but his two further relapses were marked by an increase in activity, staying out late drinking and taking drugs, spending all his money, and giving away his possessions.

Ann had been away from home in the two weeks when he had become ill prior to the last admission, and felt that she might have been able to prevent a relapse if she had been there, for example by restricting his access to money to get drugs since she felt that the marijuana brought on the relapses. She was aware of his diagnosis of schizophrenia, and had joined the local support group of the National Schizophrenia Fellowship. Ann was very distressed during her detailed account of Martin's illness history, and reported a lot of anxiety during his periods of illness and hospitalization. She wondered 'where it will all end', and felt they were going round in circles. She found his behaviour when ill difficult to cope with, but tended to try and 'persuade him out of his unreality'.

The father gave a consistent but shorter account of the illness history. He had felt under a great deal of strain when Martin's behaviour became disturbed prior to the current admission. There had been two weeks of him staying out late, sometimes all night, or staying up all night playing loud music and smoking marijuana, and bringing out of work 'hippy' types to the house. Jim had attempted to talk to Martin about his behaviour, but felt that if he said too much then Martin would have left home, and this would have caused more problems since he would have felt the need to go and find Martin because he knew he was ill. Jim was surprised that Martin seemed to lack insight into his illness, and had laughed at his father when he had tried to persuade him that he was ill again and needed to go into hospital. Martin had maintained that it was the rest of the world that was ill, and that he felt free and in contact with special powers. Jim felt that up to now he had hoped that Martin might recover, but since the last relapse now felt despondent for his prospects.

Irritability

The mother, Ann, reported that Martin was never irritable when well, and had always had an easy-going nature. There had been a couple of incidents in the past when he was acutely ill where there'd been disagreement between her and Martin, and on one of these occasions Martin had been verbally aggressive with her. The disagreements were triggered by Ann telling Martin he was spending too much money, and that she thought he ought not to spend time with people who took drugs. Ann said she felt her husband got annoyed with Martin's lack of activity in the house, but Jim tended to tell her about it rather than show Martin his annoyance.

The father agreed with his wife's comments about Martin's disposition. He said that most of the irritability in the house tended to be between himself and his wife, rather than directed at Martin. Jim felt that being unemployed made him more irritable, but that he found Martin's lethargy more difficult to cope with than his behaviour when acutely ill. Minor disagreements with his wife focused on the housework; sometimes she would start doing jobs he had already spent time doing; or Jim felt that Martin should do more, but Ann thought this was 'getting' at Martin.

Current problems/symptoms

Ann had seen little of Martin at home during his recent acute illness phase since she had been staying with her daughter. However, during his hospitalization she had become very concerned about some of his behaviours, and on one occasion during weekend leave had tried to dissuade him from going out, and had attempted to get his bank to prevent him from withdrawing money without her consent. However, such attempts to control his excesses had always failed. Ann was particularly concerned about him taking street drugs, since she felt that this brought on his relapses. He talked to himself when ill, and would sit giggling to himself, and Ann was aware that he heard voices; she also said he currently had ideas that were connected with outer-space and talked a lot about spacemen, but didn't know what this was about.

When she visited him in hospital, he often tended not to answer her when she spoke to him, and this concerned her. His appearance also concerned her; she said Martin usually looked scruffy because of his long hair, which he didn't wash very often, and his clothes, usually old jeans with holes in and baggy old jumpers. Ann expressed some dissatisfaction with his lethargy at home prior to the relapse, and the fact that he did very little housework and none at all unless prompted. His 'irresponsible' attitude to money also troubled her: she and Jim only requested a small amount from his social security benefits for rent which did not cover his keep, and they encouraged him to save money. However, he spent money on cigarettes, records or alcohol, and had 'blown' most his savings in the weeks before he was admitted to hospital. Ann felt that Martin was generally 'stubborn' and was frustrated by the fact that 'he wouldn't listen to advice'. She was concerned that unless he stopped the drugs and drinking, he would never get better. She and Jim found they had had to cut down on the money they spent since Martin was living with them, for example they were unable to go on holiday or out for meals.

The father's description of Martin's problems and symptoms was generally in agreement with his wife's. Like Ann, he was aware that Martin had hallucinations and strange ideas when ill, but did not seem to know the content of these, rather the effects on his behaviour. He also found his drug-taking and drinking very worrying, both from the point of view of money being squandered, and also its effect on Martin's relapses. He found his son's 'hippy-like' appearance embarrassing, and felt it drew attention to the fact that Martin had a mental illness. He was particularly put out by Martin's inactivity at home, and was more critical of this than his wife. He felt that Martin did have energy sometimes but put this into going to the pub rather than helping in the house, and that he was disinclined to do house-work, rather than handicapped by his illness. He didn't tell Martin of his feelings or try to get him to do more, because he didn't want to cause him stress by arguing.

Relationship with the patient
Ann was very warm in her descriptions of her relationship with Martin. She described him as a kind, intelligent, and friendly person. She said that she had felt closer to him since his illness, and that she would do anything to help him: 'I am prepared to give my life to it' (i.e. Martin's illness problems). His problems caused her great concern, and she found it difficult to get on with her own life when he was ill. She had had problems sleeping since his relapse and was taking sleeping tablets, and had difficulty concentrating at work. For her, the most upsetting part of the illness was the effects on Martin's life.

She felt his opportunities, for example to get a good job and to marry, were greatly diminished.

Jim also expressed a great deal of warmth towards Martin. He said he felt closer to Martin since his illness. He had become depressed since Martin's relapse, and felt hopeless about him ever recovering and living a normal life. He too was distressed by the deterioration in the quality of Martin's life since the illness onset.

Effects of the illness on themselves

Ann felt that Jim sometimes got jealous of the amount of time and concern she showed Martin, and they sometimes argued about this, particularly about their attitudes to Martin's inactivity in the home. However, she felt Martin came first, and that it was important that she did everything in her power to help him. She did less activities with her husband than they had shared in the past. They rarely went out socially together. This was partly due to financial constraints, and partly due to a reluctance on her part to do things which did not include Martin. Her job carried a lot of responsibility, and she had managed to continue it throughout Martin's illness, but would liked to have more time to spend with him. She had a number of friends at work, but did not socialize outside of work, other than with the family. Ann felt that this was partly due to a lack of time, but also due to the demands of Martin's problems.

Jim felt that changes in his life were partly due to Martin, and also to his unemployment. He was dissatisfied with staying at home most days, and missed the company of workmates. He occasionally went for a drink with a friend, but that was the limit of his social life outside the family. He would like to spend more time alone with Ann, but she was often tired from work and preoccupied with Martin's problems.

GHQ Assessments

Both parents scored just above the threshold for psychiatric disturbance on the General Health Questionnaire. This was consistent with their accounts of pyschological distress reported in the interviews.

Family Questionnaire

Jim identified Martin as having experienced many more of the listed items than did Ann (38 compared with 20). This could have been due in part to the fact that the father had had much more contact with Martin when he became acutely ill than did Ann, since she was away visiting her daughter. Jim, however, perceived himself to be less bothered by the problems than did Ann. He reported difficulty coping mainly with the behavioural excesses or disturbances than Martin had shown during the acute illness phase (staying out late, taking drugs, drinking, mixing with undesirable company and so on), but he rated himself as being 'not at all' able to cope with Martin's unwillingness to do housework and his odd appearance and untidiness. Ann reported that she was bothered quite a lot by most of the items that she marked, but felt able to cope with most problems.

Summary of the Parent's Problems, Needs, and Strengths (As Obtained From the Interviews, GHQ, and FQ Assessments)

Understanding the illness

Problems
Although both parents had acquired some considerable knowledge about schizophrenia over the course of the illness, there was evidence that there were still some issues they were unclear about. Taking acount of both parent's interviews these included: how much insight Martin had, or could be expected to have, about his problems when in remission and when acutely ill; the role of marijuana smoking and alcohol in relapse; the nature and content of his delusions and auditory hallucinations and how these might affect his behaviour; the nature of negative symtoms and how much control he had over his inactivity; the course of the illness and the range of possible outcomes for Martin.

Needs
Further information about the illness and its treatment.

Distress and Situations Triggering Distress

Problems
The amount of distress reported by Ann and Jim was not extreme, given that Martin had recently suffered a relapse and his behaviour at home had caused problems. However, Ann particularly suggested that her emotional well-being was closely tied to her son's behaviour, and that she was constantly preoccupied with his problems. Her general worries concerned his future, and she reported sleep disturbance and some difficulties with work as a consequence. These worries also preoccupied Jim, if to a lesser degree. Specific situations which caused anxiety included dealing with the behavioural excesses (drinking, drugs, money) when he was acutely ill. Jim and Ann were stressed by Martin's inactivity at home, which caused disagreements between the parents.

Needs
Alternative ways of coping with difficult situations when Martin is ill; further assessment of the nature of general long-term worries; help with communication and problem-solving of the inactivity issue.

Coping Strategies

Aside from the difficulties with the acute illness behaviours mentioned above, both parents indicated they felt their attempts to help Martin when in remission were not very successful.

Problems
The father reported that although annoyed and dismayed by Martin's lack of progress and inactivity, he tended not to prompt behaviours. Although the mother had made some good attempts to initiate and prompt activities for Martin, she showed some indications of 'self-sacrificing' behaviours in these attempts, with adverse effects on her own lifestyle; Martin's activities did not become self-initiating, but were dependent on her continued presence.

Needs
Help with devising and implementing alternative strategies for dealing with both acute illness behaviours and negative behaviours.

Restrictions to Lifestyles

Jim recognized that the biggest restricting factor in his own life was unemployment, and there was no evidence that his problem of being unable to get work was associated with Martin's illness: at the time of the intervention there was a very high unemployment rate in the town.

Problems
However, there were financial and social consequences to the illness which included reduced money available for outings and holidays; Jim and Ann spent little time together; Ann was mainly busy working or helping Martin and had little time for herself.

Needs
To consider the distribution of the family's finances; Jim and Ann to re-establish shared activities; Ann to re-evaluate how much time it was useful for her to spend with Martin, and to consider alternative ways of helping him.

Dissatisfactions with Martin's Behaviour

Although both parents said they usually did not openly criticize or nag Martin, it was evident from the interviews and from the FQ responses that they had a number of concerns or dissatisfactions.

Problems
Included Martin's inactivity when his illness was in remission, and particularly his father's annoyance at him not offering help in the house; his smoking marijuana and drinking alcohol to excess; his money management; his scruffy appearance.

Needs
Assistance with helping Martin to change his behaviours, or help for the parents in coping with the problems.

Strengths

These included both parents having a good relationship with their son, and were very keen to work with the therapist on the family programme; there was evidence that some coping strategies had already been tried, even if these had not been entirely successful; the other siblings were also keen to help; the parents had some considerable knowledge about the illness and support from the Schizophrenia Fellowship; the mother had continued with her busy and demanding job, despite the problems at home.

We have found that the above format of problems and needs – summarized under key headings, with a note on the family's strengths – is an extremely useful way of summarizing the situation. The focus on needs shifts the emphasis of the assessment away from family deficits and focuses on directions for positive change, so the rationale behind interventions becomes evident. Moreover, the interventions do not seek to eradicate problems but rather to help formulate and meet the needs of the family, using and acknowledging whatever resources they have available.

Although the problems have been categorized under headings, it is apparent there is a lot of overlap between categories. For example, sources of distress are also coping difficulties, and may arise from lack of understanding about the illness. The function of the summary is to clarify areas of need and to feed these back to the relative, and to indicate the directions of assistance the intervention might take: success in one aspect of intervention may well facilitate change in another area, or meet more than one of the relative's needs. At this stage, needs are only outlined in general terms: specific details and behavioural goals will be worked out as the intervention progresses.

THE PATIENT'S ASSESSMENT

As with the relatives, the aim of the patient's assessment is to identify problems and strengths so that areas of need may be ascertained. Three broad assessment themes will be important for the intervention components: firstly, psychopathology of current (if first seen during acute episode) and past illness episodes; whether some psychotic symptoms are resistant to medication; medication history and compliance. Secondly, the patient's level of functioning, including behavioural excesses and deficits, both currently and over the course of the illness. Thirdly, the patient's strengths, e.g., interests, abilities, supports, resources.

If possible, the patient should be interviewed and similar content areas discussed as are described in the RAI. In this way a chronological account of the illness might be obtained from the patient; their report of past and particularly current symptomatology sought, and how it has affected or continues to affect everyday activities; details of how the illness has affected their life generally; and the nature of any problems in the family or community contexts discussed.

In practice, long interviews and detailed questioning of the patient may be impossible, particularly when the patient is acutely ill or actively psychotic. It may be necessary to rely on information given by the relatives, or from other professionals, from the case-notes, and whatever brief assessments with the patient are possible. Assessment scales or forms are helpful for the systematic collection of information. Useful measures are described below.

Symptomatology Scales

A number of scales can be used for assessing current symptomatology. For example, the Psychiatric Assessment Scales (PAS) (Krawiecka *et al.*, 1977), which measure anxiety, depression, hallucinations, delusions, incoherence and irrelevance of speech, poverty of speech, flat or incongruous affect, and psychomotor retardation on a five-point scale (0=absent, and 4=extremely severe), which are useful for evaluating change in symptoms over time. It is suitable for use only by a clinician who knows the patient well. An alternative is the use of appropriate scales from the BPRS (Lukoff *et al.*, 1986).

It is advisable that the patient's clinical state is monitored throughout the intervention, in order to inform relatives of how the patient's behaviour may be affected by current symptoms, as well as to evaluate the patient's progress and to evaluate intervention outcomes.

Social Functioning Scales (SFS)

The SFS (Appendix 3) (Birchwood *et al.*, 1990) is recommended since it has several advantages over other available scales of social adjustment. It may be completed using the relative(s) as informant, and covers seven areas of social functioning: social engagement/withdrawal; interpersonal behaviour; prosocial activities; recreation, independence in living skills (compentence and performance); and employment/occupation. Since it provides a detailed assessment of the patient's strengths and weaknesses, the SFS can be a helpful guide to possible intervention goals, as well as a measure of progress and outcome.

Other useful assessments include the Personal Functioning Scales (Appendix 4), which were designed by the authors to be completed by relatives as a repeated measure (every month, or at other set intervals) for assessing the patient's behaviour in the home context.

EVALUATING INTERVENTION OUTCOMES

The efficacy of family interventions needs to be assessed through the use of multiple-outcome measures. This applies not just to large-scale controlled studies, but is also important for single-case clinical interventions. As with any other cognitive-behavioural approach, it is important that progress and outcomes are validated by reliable and objective measures.

These measures might include repeated assessments of targeted variables, such as relatives' well-being, or concern about patient problems; or patient symptomatology, relapse or social functioning, using some of the assessment scales, forms, and questionnaires suggested in this chapter; as well as the ongoing evaluation of progress by monitoring targets for change, or the achievement of operationalized goals which are set during the intervention. Diaries and record forms also can be devized for such purposes (Chapters 6 and 7).

CONCLUSION

At the end of the initial assessments, the therapist should have formed a broad picture about the patient's illness in terms of the symptoms, behaviours, and responses to treatment; and an understanding of how the relatives have coped with the problems associated with the patient's illness, and what are their current chief concerns and difficulties in the home situation.

The chapter was written with the therapist who has had no previous contact with the family in mind. For therapists who already know the patient or his/her family well, and have established a good relationship with the relatives, some of the assessment procedures described may be unnecessary. Similarly, it may be more appropriate to adapt existing assessment measures that are already used rather than to repeat assessments in a rigid adherence to the guidelines presented here.

The next three chapters describe the three main intervention components: education about the illness; stress management, including coping stategies; and goal-setting for patient behaviour change. These are broad areas for intervention work with the family.

The needs assessments that have been collected will provide the background to the nature of the interventions implemented. For example, some of the key issues of misunderstanding about the illness should be apparent and will inform your educational work; situations which trigger stress responses and coping problems may be apparent and can be targeted for intervention; and the areas of patient functioning which present problems may be appropriate for change through goal-setting. However, we should emphasize to those who are not familiar with cognitive-behavioural approaches that further assessment continues to be an integral part of the intervention process. Thus, the description of each component of intervention begins with how further assessments may be conducted, and how such assessments feed into the intervention process.

Working with families of schizophrenic patients does not involve the delivery of standard packages of treatment. Although the needs of relatives are sufficiently uniform to permit us to organize intervention strategies along three main themes or components, it should be emphasized that firstly, these components should not be seen as discrete or time limited, for example, giving relatives information about schizophrenia does not end when the education component has been delivered to the relatives; secondly, the aim of the interventions is to address the needs of the family. Accordingly, with each family some components or intervention aspects will be much more important than others, for example, where relatives are experiencing very high levels of distress and/or where the patient is severely handicapped by unremitting psychotic symptoms, it may be more appropriate to concentrate on helping the relative to manage their distress and to cope with difficult patient behaviours than to set goals aimed at directly changing patient behaviour. Thirdly, working with relatives to address their needs and improve patient functioning may be only one intervention from the total range of services available to the patient and his or her family. Thus it is important to communicate assessments and plans with members of the larger multidisciplinary team who are involved with the patient's treatment and support.

Chapter 5

Education

This chapter sets out advice on the form and content that educative components with family members might take. Since information-giving to relatives has been the subject of considerable discussion and analysis, the first part of the chapter reviews some of the pertinent issues. An understanding of the complexities of helping consumers to better understand the schizophrenic illness, and an appreciation of the interactive nature of the process, are important in assisting therapists to carry out individualized and effective programmes.

BENEFITS AND LIMITATIONS OF EDUCATION COMPONENTS

Although family education was a common component in the major long-term family intervention studies, its specific role was unclear (Smith *et al.*, 1987), and its evaluation was limited. Increases in relatives' knowledge about schizophrenia following the education were reported (McGill *et al.*, 1983; Berkowitz *et al.*, 1984; Barrowclough *et al.*, 1987), however, the consequences of such knowledge acquisition were largely unassessed.

We know from the Salford Study that the education component alone did not reduce EE levels or relapse rates (Tarrier *et al.*, 1988a). We may deduce from this that the provision of information *per se* is unlikely to result in changing relatives' attitudes and behaviours, at least in the long-term. However, Smith and Birchwood's (1987) study in Birmingham looked at a wider number of variables and found no changes in the patient's symptomatology or disturbance, but there were improvements in the relatives' well-being, and a reduction of their fear of the patient, albeit these changes were not maintained at a six-month follow up. The authors suggested that brief educational components may best serve in facilitating a more receptive attitude to longer-term interventions for changing patient management. Thus, although the acquisition of knowledge may have limited long-term effects on patient or relative behaviours, information has an important role in setting the scene for work with families.

MODELS OF INFORMATION-GIVING

Deficit and interaction models of information-giving in relation to schizophrenia are helpful in understanding why the knowledge components *per se* are limited, and how their delivery is important if we are to maximize their value in terms of engaging relatives' cooperation.

The basic premise of the simple deficit model is that lack of information plays a causative role in producing attitudes and behaviours in relatives that have a detrimental effect on patients; providing relevant information will eliminate the knowledge deficit, and result in more beneficial attitudes and behaviours. This was the thinking behind the inclusion of the education component in the early intervention studies based on the high-EE concept. Vaughn and Leff (1981) reported that relatives who were rated high EE tended to view the bizarre and difficult behaviour of the patient as being deliberate or at least controllable; low-EE relatives believed this behaviour was due to a legitimate illness which the patient was not able to control. Thus Berkowitz *et al.* (1984) comment on the inclusion of the intervention component in Leff *et al.*'s (1982) study:

> The reasoning was that if high EE relatives could learn more about schizophrenia, they might begin to understand that some of the patient's bizarre or difficult behaviour could be attributed to the schizophrenic condition. Such understanding could be one of the apparently important changes necessary for the change from low to high EE.

The second, more complex, model – interaction – is suggested by Tarrier and Barrowclough (1986) to be more appropriate for conceptualizing the information-giving process than the deficit approach. This highlights the distinction between disease and illness, the former being a medical paradigm and referring to 'objective' pathology, whereas the latter refers to the 'subjective' effects of the patient having the disease.

Lay people develop their own subjective models of illness in order to make sense of ill health, and these will influence the assimilation of any new information offered to them. The use of lay models of sickness by the patient and relatives is likely to occur in psychiatric illness, where symptoms are seen in terms of changes in behaviour, and not as physical signs of pathology. What the psychiatrist terms a 'persecutory delusion' may be manifest to the relative in patient behaviours such as hiding indoors behind closed curtains, or verbal and physical assaults on family members. Even though the relative might 'learn' that delusions are key symptoms of schizophrenia, they may retain a model of the patient's problems based on ideas that the behaviours are caused by events such as those that occurred in childhood, and that, for example, the patient elects to live in a fantasy world rather than facing up to reality, and is angry and jealous of more successful siblings.

It is suggested that the health care professional usually assumes a disease model of schizophrenia, whereas the family will hold individualized illness models. Such illness models may result in shaping the management strategies that relatives adopt, and as such play a significant role in helping the relative cope with and control the negative and distressing consequences of the illness. There is some evidence that relatives engage in a good deal of causal searching as to why symptoms or behaviours occur, and it is likely that their responses to the patient are mediated by the kinds of answers they form.

Information given by others will be assimilated, organized, and possibly rejected on the basis of the illness model held by the relative, even if they adopt the medical terminology presented; changing the relatives' model may well require giving them detailed help as to how this new way of looking at the illness translates into more effective management strategies. Thus the model adopted by the therapist – deficit or interaction – will direct how information is communicated, and may affect the satisfaction, compliance, and receptiveness for change of the relative. It is argued that an interactional style that acknowledges and respects the relative's existing illness model is the most appropriate in working with the family. This is likely to be most pertinent in families where the patient's illness is chronic, and the relatives have developed individual illness models and methods of coping with the disturbed behaviours of the patient over years, and largely without professional resources. There is some evidence that information is more readily assimilated and illness models changed by relatives of more recent onset patients (Barrowclough *et al.*, 1987), and that in such cases brief education combined with some advice on management strategies can reduce relapse in first episode patients (Goldstein *et al.*, 1981).

OTHER ASPECTS OF INFORMATION PRESENTATION

Working in service settings, where there are heavy demands on staff time and resources, it is important to consider whether therapist presentation of information has advantages over less staff-time intensive methods. In reported educational programmes, the method of information delivery has varied considerably in terms of whether it is presented to individual relatives, to the family-patient unit, or to groups of relatives, and whether in the form of lectures, oral presentations with discussion, or written booklets (Tarrier *et al.*, 1986; Birchwood *et al.*, in press).

Birchwood, Smith, and colleagues have evaluated the specific (knowledge gained) and non-specific (e.g., symptoms of stress and perceived burden) effects of different forms of information delivery. They compared information given by therapists in group situations, with written-booklet form only, and video presentations. Although the therapist-present condition resulted in most information being acquired, in the longer term this did not hold any advantage over the other two formats. All formats led to gains in assessed knowledge, increased optimism concerning the family's role in treatment, and reductions in relatives' stress symptoms at six-months' follow up.

This suggests that interventions that are limited to brief educational components alone may have some benefits to families, and that receiving written information only, or that supplemented with a video, may not be detrimental to information uptake, although some relatives expressed a preference for having a therapist available to clarify points and discuss issues. Thus it would be good practice – without being detrimental to information uptake or relatives' well-being – to have available information videos and booklets, perhaps in the hospital ward or community health centre. As Birchwood and colleagues point out, this may sometimes be the only means available for conveying information to relatives, particularly when it is not possible for some family members to attend appointments.

Despite the benefits of short-education packages, however, assisting relatives to, on the one hand, acquire a high level of knowledge about schizophrenia, and, on the other, to use the knowledge in management strategies are two different goals. How well relatives are subsequently able to apply the knowledge gained from brief interventions to their own domestic circumstances by changing their perceptions of patient behaviour and their coping strategies has not been assessed. The evidence suggests that brief education is insufficient to change relatives' behaviour and have an effect on patient outcome; and we have underlined the importance of understanding relatives' individual models of the illness as a starting point for changing their beliefs and behaviours. This involves individualized rather than general assessments of knowledge, which are considered in later sections of the chapter.

Before leaving the discussion of presentation format, it is worth making some further points about relatives' comprehension of information. Attention should be given to the reading level required for any written materials distributed, and a reading analysis (Flesch, 1948) should be performed on materials which have not previously been assessed. Relatively simple language expression is necessary if the content is to be understood by most of the general population. Next, research into doctor-patient communication suggests that only a few items of information can be retained by recipients (Ley, 1979), making it necessary to be selective in the information presented. Finally, it should not be assumed that everyone will assimilate the information at the same rate.

GENERAL CONCLUSIONS

On the basis of the preceding discussions and research evidence, some general conclusions about giving information to relatives can be derived.

Brief educational input can have a valuable role. Studies show that relatives are able to retain at least part of the information presented, and that there are also gains in terms of relatives' well-being, particularly in the short term. Even written or video presentations of information without discussion and clarification from staff are beneficial. However, such brief interventions do not seem to have an effect on the course of the illness, and this suggests they do not change the management practices of relatives. In long-term interventions with families, the education component may best be construed as helping to prepare relatives for changing their behaviour.

Where changing relatives' behaviour is the goal, there is a need to assess relatives' perceptions of the illness before giving further information. We advocate the adoption of the interaction model, whereby we assume the relative already holds some beliefs about the cause and maintenance of the symptoms, as well as views on treatments and how behaviours are best managed at home.

It is important to accept the individualized illness model, which involves taking the views of the relatives seriously, while presenting alternative explanations and ways of coping. It also involves focusing on the symptoms and behaviours particular to the patient, and how these present in the domestic environment, rather than imparting general academic knowledge. Beliefs that are helpful in mediating management strategies and are likely to have a beneficial effect on the course of the illness are those to be encouraged; conversely, those ideas which may lead to relative behaviours with potentially detrimental effects on the patient's condition are those we need to target for change.

We should not overload the relatives with information; make written materials accessible to them; and expect everyone to assimilate information at a uniform rate.

The interaction model predicts that the longer the duration of the illness, the more time and opportunity there has been for a personalized, lay model of the illness to become established, especially where no professional view has been offered. Consequently, the sooner information is given after the illness begins, the greater its influence is likely to be on relatives' beliefs.

PRACTICAL GUIDELINES FOR CONDUCTING EDUCATION SESSIONS

We have acknowledged the usefulness of education programmes *per se*, but limit the process described here to giving information in the context of a long-term family intervention, and to working with individual families rather than groups. However, practitioners embarking on brief-education formats with individuals or groups may find some of the advice and discussion useful.

On the basis of our discussion of the literature cited, the educational component would be seen as the entry into a working partnership with the family, and assisting to engage the family members in treatment. Many relatives have been told very little about the illness, and most regard access to detailed information about schizophrenia as a need of high priority. The education sessions also serve to present the theoretical framework or rationale in which other work with the family will take place. This rationale emphasizes that schizophrenia is a stress-related, biological illness influenced in its course by the social environment: the family members are in no way to blame for having caused the illness, and on the contrary are an important resource in assisting in the patient's recovery. On the same theme, it allows us to assess the relatives' perceptions about the illness, to find out how their beliefs influence their behaviour, and how amenable they are to seeing things from a different viewpoint.

ASSESSMENTS PRIOR TO GIVING INFORMATION

Information-giving should be preceded by taking stock of what has been found out about the relative's understanding of the illness in the RAI, and organizing further assessments.

Relative Assessments

We have emphasized that an understanding of the relatives' beliefs and attitudes about the illness in general, and the symptoms of the patient in particular, is a necessary precondition establishing an interactive mode of information presentation. Information from the initial interviews will be useful to this understanding, and it may be helpful to collect more detailed information using, for example, the Knowledge About Schizophrenia Interview (KASI) (Barrowclough *et al.*, 1987; Appendix 5). The KASI aims to assess and evaluate and relative's information, beliefs, and attitudes about six broad aspects of the illness:

1. **Diagnosis** What kind of problem does the relative think the patient is being treated for?
2. **Symptomatology** Does the relative believe the 'key' symptoms, such as the relative him/herself has identified in the RAI, are part of the illness, or personality related? Is he relative aware of florid symptoms (hallucinations and delusions)? Do they understand that negative symptoms are features of the illness?
3. **Aetiology** What caused the illness according to the relative?
4. **Medication** Is the relative aware of the long-term and prophylactic nature of the medication?
5. **Prognosis** Does the relative accept the possibility of recurrence, and what does he/she think might cause relapse?
6. **Management** What does the relative think he/she should or should not do to assist the patient's recovery?

The relative's responses can be evaluated in terms of how helpful or unhelpful the beliefs they hold are likely to be to the management of the patient. (Scoring the KASI, based on the value of beliefs to the management of the illness, is contained in Appendix 5.)

The interview should take 10–30 minutes to administer, depending on the relative's length of response and the therapist's ability to structure the interview; or it can be incorporated into the RAI. It should, of course, be used in a conversational manner, and not presented as a test with right and wrong answers.

Patient Assessments

It is advisable to have a detailed knowledge of the patient's past and present psychopathology, which should be available from your initial assessments of the patient. Knowledge of the content of their delusions, nature of hallucinations, behaviours related to these symptoms (e.g., the belief that a TV broadcasting their thoughts is associated with the refusal to enter the TV room, or the smashing of the TV set), negative symptoms, and variation in symptoms across episodes of acute illness will be helpful in providing the relatives with a personalized viewpoint of the illness.

Questions that need to be considered include: is the patient aware of the diagnosis? Do they accept that they have a mental illness? Do they have any objections to disclosing details of their symptoms to their wife, mother, father, or other relatives? In the latter, the confidentiality of aspects of the patient's symptoms needs to be considered. For a number of patients the delusions they held when acutely ill may cause them embarrassment when they have more insight into their illness, for example, if delusions were of a sexual nature, and it can never be assumed that the patient would wish the content of their preoccupations to be discussed with family members.

Format

If there is more than one key relative, a useful format for information-giving is to assess the relatives' existing level of knowledge in short individual sessions or as part of the RAI, and then to present information to the family collectively.

There are no hard-and-fast rules as to when and how to include the patient in the sessions: factors such as the age of the patient, their relationship to the relative, and their current level of functioning may influence such decisions. A parallel but separate information-giving session for the patient is often useful, with their attendance at the end of the relatives' session, or at a later session with the rest of the family. In the first instance, allowing the relatives to see the therapist without the patient present may be preferable: there are often questions the relative wants to raise, which they would feel uncomfortable talking about if the patient were there, for example, 'Will she ever work again?' 'Will he ever recover?', as well as issues of guilt or embarrassment about the problems.

One of the benefits of having the patient attend the later discussion of the illness with the relatives can be the communication of feelings and thoughts the patient experienced during the illness, if they are comfortable talking about these matters. The relatives only see behavioural correlates of florid symptoms, and may be unaware of the thinking and fears behind seemingly impulsive and bizarre behaviours. However, not all patients will be able or willing to communicate their experiential symptoms, and some patients may disrupt the sessions when, for example, they are only able to sit for short periods, or their speech is disturbed, or they are unable to concentrate, or show inappropriate affect.

The education component of the intervention may involve two or more initial sessions.

Session One

The first session consists of presentation and discussion of information with the relatives together, paying particular attention to misunderstandings about the illness. Some of the guidelines of what are, on the one hand, 'helpful beliefs/information', and, on the other hand, 'unhelpful beliefs information' for aspects of the illness are given later. These descriptive guidelines summarize the KASI scoring criteria. If it is the patient's first episode of schizophrenia, some of the issues need special consideration, for example the likelihood of future episodes or relapses.

During the session, discussion should refer frequently to the relatives' assessed beliefs about the condition, for example:

'When we were talking earlier, you mentioned that you felt that Peter stayed in bed too much, and you wondered whether this was due to his medication or because he was lazy. Another explanation could be the illness itself. Some of the symptoms of the illness are called negative symptoms. These symptoms include difficulty in doing ordinary things, and it is quite common that people want to sleep or to lie around more than usual.'

Acceptance of the relative's viewpoint while suggesting alternative explanations is the starting point of changing the relatives' 'unhelpful' beliefs, and engaging them in a more positive approach to the management of patient difficulties. Care should be taken not to overload the relative with too much information or medical jargon. The aim is to help the relatives to acquire information likely to have a beneficial influence on their interactions with the patient, rather than to learn academic or technical knowledge.

As mentioned, it is useful to see the relatives and the patient together for the latter part of the session, and, if appropriate, the patient can be encouraged to describe the thinking which directed his or her actions during periods of acute illness and disturbed behaviour. A short interval between the first education session and follow-up is advisable, during which time the family is asked to read an information booklet covering the material presented in the session (Appendix 6). Relatives occasionally become worried or misunderstand information once they have left the therapist; an early second appointment provides an opportunity for discussion of such difficulties.

Therapists may be concerned that they do not know enough about the illness to provide answers to all the relatives' questions. Honesty is the best policy, and an admission of uncertainty about points raised, with the assurance of seeking out information for the next session, has always been acceptable to relatives in our experience. However, we would advise that therapists ensure they are comfortable in their general knowledge about the illness, and particularly as it pertains to the individual patient (Chapters 3 and 4; Further Reading). Some relatives will seek out further reading, and its better that they are directed to sources concordant with the approach the therapist is taking, rather than taking chances at the local library. Some common questions, with discussion of how they might be answered can be found in Appendix 7.

Session Two

At the second appointment, relatives and patient may be seen together, and further discussion prompted. The therapist should actively encourage the relatives to consider any problems they have in assimilating explanations about the illness and its treatment which differ from those previously held. For example, 'When we talked earlier, you said you were worried your daughter might get addicted to the medication and would be better off without it. What do you think about that now?' A post-test of knowledge using the KASI following this session is useful in assessing areas where further attitude or belief change will be important, since it is unlikely that relatives, particularly where patients have a long history of illness, will change all their views after a brief educational component.

The goal of the sessions described is to prepare the ground for change, and to assess problem areas rather than to 'complete' the education of the relative. Information-giving and continuous assessment of the views of the relative, and how these relate to their interactions with the patient and the services are continuing and essential components of the intervention.

CONCLUSION

We should again emphasize that informing relatives about schizophrenic illness is a continuing process, and that the brief introduction to the information and ideas we have described is best viewed as laying the groundwork for further collaboration between relatives and therapists. In our experience and from research findings, we know that although the majority of relatives will benefit in terms of increasing their knowledge of the illness and improving their well-being from short educational interventions, some relatives will remember very little information and retain their own beliefs about the illness. We have discussed some of the reasons why this might be the case in earlier sections of this chapter. We certainly met several relatives who totally rejected all new information: one mother of a man with a long illness history announced at the second education session, 'I don't know who wrote that booklet you gave me, but they know nothing about schizophrenia!' A more common response was for relatives to accept some new information, but to retain some of their own beliefs as well, especially when the illness was longstanding.

One of the values of the educational component, especially if it has been conducted in the interactional style which we recommend, is that the therapist will gain considerable understanding of the relative's viewpoint, and will know what beliefs might continue to maintain the relative's worries and concerns, or interfere with the implementation of more effective coping strategies. The examples in the next few chapters will highlight these points, and will demonstrate the need for a continuing educational input for many families.

Chapter 6

Stress Management and Coping Responses

This component of the intervention focuses primarily on the needs of the relatives; its aim is to reduce the levels of reported distress by the use of cognitive behavioural approaches. Stress-management techniques have been extensively used to help people to cope with a wide variety of problems and conditions. The authors are not offering a new approach, but rather aim to demonstrate how stress management can be used in the context of families of schizophrenic patients. Although for the purposes of this book the procedures and techniques are compartmentalized, we emphasize that teaching people to improve their coping responses to stressful situations is a continuing process.

Following the assessment of situations presenting difficulties to relatives and the education sessions, a more fine-grained assessment of individual difficulties is conducted, leading to the development of ways of responding to problems more effectively. This chapter details how such assessments may be conducted, and outlines the principles of stress reduction, with reference to examples presented by families in our clinical experience.

WHAT DO WE MEAN BY STRESS?

'Stress' is a term that is used extensively but often imprecisely in work with schizophrenic patients, both in terms of the effect of psychosocial stress on the patient, and the stress experienced by relatives as a result of living with someone who has a mental illness. Our focus here is on the latter use of the term. It is worthwhile considering how such stress is usefully conceptualized. The following case example examines the nature of stressful events associated with mental illness in the family environment.

Case Example

Anne Fleming is the mother of an 18-year-old daughter, Jane, who was discharged from psychiatric hospital three months ago after what was described by the psychiatrist as a schizophrenic breakdown. The illness has caused the family considerable upset. The onset was fairly sudden, although looking back Jane had had difficulties with college work for some time, and had become increasingly withdrawn and reluctant to go out with friends. For the two-week period before she went into hospital, the parents had been at a loss to know what to do: Jane had refused to eat, had become distressed when the TV was on, had accused the neighbours of trying to kill her, and had become fearful of her father, who she claimed was an imposter. After treatment with medication in hospital, she had shown much improvement, and after a couple of months at home, the psychiatrist had suggested she go back to college to complete her 'A' levels. Jane had wanted this herself, and the college was supportive. The problem was getting Jane up and off to college in the morning.

This was the second month of Mrs Fleming's attempt to get Jane up in time to get the 8.30 bus. The first week had not been too much of a problem, but by the second week difficulties arose. Despite the mother's attempts to persuade her to get up, Jane frequently did not rise until lunchtime, and more often than not did not go into college at all. Mrs Fleming had to leave the house at 10 a.m. to go to her part-time job. Mr Fleming was often away on business during the week, and the other daughter was living in another town while at university.

On the Monday morning Mrs Fleming was feeling tired and anxious. Jane had spent most of the weekend in bed. Anne Fleming and her husband had had lengthy discussions about what to do about this, and whether they should persevere in trying to get Jane to college. Mr Fleming thought they should leave the decision to Jane. Jane said she wanted to go, and Mrs Fleming said that was all very well, but what about trying to get up in the morning? Mrs Fleming had spent the night worrying about what Jane would do if she did not continue with college, and had become upset when she contrasted how her daughter had been before the illness to her present state. Jane no longer seemed interested in her appearance, did not want to see her friends, and when her grandmother visited had left the room saying she was tired.

At 7.30 a.m. Mrs Fleming called Jane. By 8 a.m. there was no response, so she went into the room and started reasoning with her daughter, saying how important it was to start getting up if she was to get her bus. Jane said she would get up, but ten minutes later there was no movement. Mrs Fleming felt irritated. She went in and pulled the bedclothes off, and said that if she did not get up now, then not to expect her to bother trying again. Jane said that was fine by her, but she felt too tired to move and would go in on a later bus. Jane had not stirred when her mother left for work. In fact, it was apparent that she had only just got up when her mother returned home at 4 p.m. Mrs Fleming had been worrying most of the day, and had an argument with Jane on her return.

In this example, stress can be looked at in a number of ways. Firstly, there is stress as a stimulus or trigger. The mother can be seen to be under a considerable amount of stress arising from her daughter's illness and its behavioural consequences. In the acute phase, her daughter's disturbed behaviours were stressful, and latterly there is the stress of her daughter's failure to get up. Secondly, there is stress as a response. Given the changes in her daughter's behaviour and her difficulties in getting to college and continuing her previously purposeful life, the mother is experiencing stress responses – worry, anxiety, sleep problems, arguments – when her attempts to help her daughter fail.

It is generally argued that stress is best seen as a transaction between the stimulus – in this case, the illness and its consequences – and the individual's response – attempts to cope. When people feel unable to cope with problems or difficulties, or their coping attempts do not resolve the problems, they can be said to experience stress, or stress responses become apparent.

The transactional model is important for conceptualizing how it is possible to intervene to help relatives, and how it may be used as part of the rationale for interventions. Without denying the very real triggers of stress, the model underlines the importance of the individual's reactions in determining stress responses: how the relative construes situations and what they do about them may serve to maintain stress responses which do not resolve problems and make the relative feel worse. In the example given, the mother is behaving in a fairly normal way to very unusual events: most parents would be concerned about such difficulties presenting in a teenage daughter, and discussion, prompts, and persuasions might usually resolve the problem. Given the consequences and constraints of a severe mental illness, however, the problems are not resolved, and the mother becomes increasingly distressed. It should be emphasized that frequently relatives of schizophrenic patients do not need help because they are bad at coping; rather, the particular problems presented make exceptional demands on people's ability to cope, and thus stress responses are more likely to occur.

EMPHASES OF STRESS REDUCTION: THE IMPORTANCE OF FLEXIBILITY

'Any stress management training programme must be diverse and flexible . . . coping is neither a single act nor a static process.' (Meichenbaum, 1985).

In reviewing the literature on stress management and coping, Meichenbaum notes that there is no one-to-one relationship between the use of any one form of coping and adaptational outcome. This is particularly true for relatives of schizophrenic patients. Although common themes may be selected from relatives' accounts of problems and solutions, it is evident that situations precipitating stress responses are diverse, and implementation of the same strategies in different circumstances may have positive outcomes for one family, and no effect, or even negative outcomes, for another.

In deciding how best to help the family members, it is helpful to look at stress-reduction techniques as having two forms. Using the transactional model, the behaviours of the patients may be viewed to trigger stress responses in the relatives, but how the relative appraises and responds to the problems will play an important role in maintaining their own distress. It follows that there are two possible avenues to reducing the stress response. Firstly, ameliorating the problem itself through interventions would decrease or eradicate the patient's problem behaviour. Some such interventions might be independent of the relative's response, for example, medication changes that would directly affect the illness symptoms; supervision and monitoring of medication by health workers; a reduction in the time the patient spends in the house with the relative, for example, by organizing some form of day-centre attendance; or by helping the patient directly through psychological approaches to symptom management. Others types of intervention might involve the relative more directly, for example by the relative prompting the patient to engage in alternative behaviours. The second method is to help the relative to manage negative emotions, thoughts, and behaviours associated with or triggered by the patient's problems. Interventions might include helping the relative to relax, to use self-calming statements, to reappraise the patient's behaviour, to increase the time spent on their own interests.

Where there is more than one relative living with the patient, many individual stress reactions need to be understood in the nature of the wider social context in which they occur. In our own experience, most of the work will involve both problem-based coping – designed to manage the problem causing the distress – and emotion-focused coping – targeted at self-management of affect and behaviour. Because of the interactive nature of the patient and relative behaviours, changing one will often lead to improvement of the other. However, the particular needs of the family will sometimes direct an emphasis to one or other method of help.

Some of the aspects of the particular family situation that should be taken into account in selecting intervention methods include the following:

Patient or Illness Factors

Given the nature of the patient's illness, symptoms, and treatment, and the particular concerns of the relative, what are the chances of directly changing the patient's behaviour through short-term interventions? Are environmental factors – including the behaviour of the relatives – contributing to the problem behaviours that the relative is concerned about?

Relative or Family Factors

What strategies and resources has the relative available to them? What role have cognitions, affect, and behaviour in causing or maintaining difficulties? Is the relative significantly depressed, or suffering from generalized anxiety? What is the social context of the problems, and how does the behaviour of different family members contribute to the problem; in particular, is there evidence that the relative is employing coercive or intrusive methods of controlling problems?

A couple of examples may help to clarify these points:

1. The patient is a 30-year-old man, whose behaviour has been extremely disturbed for the past ten years. Although there are periods of improvement and the nature of his fears change over time, he has continued to have persecutory delusions and auditory hallucinations. He lives alone with his elderly mother, who is socially isolated. There are no other relatives locally, and the mother is financially restricted and has health and mobility problems. His mother highlights her son's tirades against imagined persecutors, currently policemen, social security officials, and health workers, as the source of much of her fear and anxiety.

Patient Factors Considered

Despite careful control of his medication, this man's positive symptoms continued and his preoccupation with 'persecutory' officials had been evident in the hospital and other settings outside his home. He had little insight into the nature of his illness, and refused to attend such day-care as was available. He was unable to participate directly in work with the therapists since this triggered his persecutory concerns, and he worried that the therapists were working against him.

Relative Factors

The patient's mother was generally anxious and significantly depressed. She had few resources available to her in terms of social support or accessible interests outside the home, and had been unable to find ways of reducing her distress. Her response to his frequent and undeniably disturbing delusional talk was a mixture of attempts to reason with him, angry confrontations, and open distress.

Emphasis of Stress Management

The son's behaviour did not seem amenable to direct change, and there was a large affective and cognitive component in his mother's response which was making her feel considerably worse without resolving the problem. It was decided to focus on reducing her anxiety response by teaching her ways of controlling her anxiety, including reappraising her son's behaviour in terms of its causes and consequences, and helping her to build up coping resources in terms of interests and activities inside and outside the home.

2. The patient is a 30-year-old man who lives with his parents and a younger sibling. He has had three acute episodes of schizophrenia, and is currently free of positive symptoms but does little at home, spending long periods lying on the bed. His father gets very angry about his lack of activity, and there are family disagreements triggered by the issue.

Patient Factors

The man was receptive to help from the therapists, had insight into his illness, and felt bored and underachieving at home, though constrained by both feelings of lethargy and underactivity. He was concerned by his family's response to his behaviour, and willing to discuss solutions.

Relative Factors

The father felt he was helping his son by trying to get him to be more active, and felt frustrated that his attempts were not succeeding. The younger son complained that the patient did less than him in terms of household jobs; the father felt his wife should do more to encourage the patient rather than doing things for him; and the mother felt her husband's nagging was making the son worse.

Emphasis of Stress Management

Attempting to directly change the son's behaviour through his co-operation and discussion, and the use of agreed prompts from his family and scheduling of activities; changing the father's appraisal of the son's behaviour by more discussion about the nature of negative symptoms; attempting to improve the family's communication and problem-solving skills.

We would like to emphasize by contrasting these examples that there are no cookbook solutions to helping to reduce stress in families. Successful interventions are dependent on a careful analysis of the individual situation. The following sections provide guidelines for assessing the nature of the relatives' individual difficulties; demonstrate how such assessments are used to formulate interventions to reduce relatives' stress; and describe some of the intervention techniques, illustrating the methods with case examples.

PRESENTING THE RATIONALE FOR STRESS MANAGEMENT AND AN OUTLINE OF THE PROGRAMME

In introducing work on stress reduction to families, it is important that the therapist has a clear idea of the rationale, and is able to communicate this to the relatives. From empirical and clinical evidence, many families living with schizophrenic patients report high levels of personal distress. Thus interventions aimed at helping relatives to appraise and cope with problems more effectively may go someway in reducing the burden of care.

The benefits to the patient can be argued on two levels. Firstly, adopting the model of the patient's vulnerability to socio-environmental stress, the empirical evidence suggests that reductions in stress in relatives and more effective coping will improve the patient's chances of relapse. Secondly, relatives may be better able to help the patient directly through rehabilitative programmes in the domestic environment if their own personal distress has been reduced.

These rationales should be clearly communicated to the relatives when the stress management component is introduced. As some relatives may misguidedly think the focus on their own behaviour implies that they are to blame for the illness, or that they are not coping as well as they might (the education component may have made such ideas apparent), care should be taken not to reinforce these ideas. The rationale might emphasize the following points:

1. Living with a person who suffers from schizophrenia can be very difficult, and it is usual for relatives to feel stressed or upset at least some of the time.
2. When the patient is living with the family, a lot of the day-to-day help and rehabilitation is carried out by family members. Hence it is important to make sure they have help in managing their own stress and coping with difficult situations if they are to help the patient effectively.
3. People who suffer from schizophrenia are unusually sensitive to stress in others; by feeling more in control of themselves, the relative may indirectly help the patient.

Care should be taken in communicating this last point lest the relative misinterprets the psychosocial stress model as a suggestion that they are making the patient worse: the positive benefits of stress reduction, rather than the negative impact on patients of stress in relatives, should be emphasized. In our experience, by helping relatives to understand something of the importance of social environments in schizophrenia, one is more likely to correct erroneous views than to plant seeds of self-blame. If the therapist fails to inform the relatives, they may pick up distorted versions of EE research and feel misled by the therapist, who has a 'hidden agenda'. A more common problem, and one to which the therapist should be sensitive, is one relative blaming the other for 'causing the patient stress', particularly in the case of parental homes. Eliciting feedback from the relatives as to what they think of the rationales can be useful, as well as illustrating the points with examples given by the relatives at previous sessions.

It is important to give the relatives a broad outline of what the programme will entail, so the relatives have some idea of what they are agreeing to. The therapist then has the opportunity to emphasize the collaborative nature of the work, which might be along the lines of the following:

'What I would like us to do is first spend some time talking about situations and concerns that cause difficulty to you and/or other members of your family. I've already heard some of the problems and solutions you've encountered from our earlier talks and the forms you filled in, but it would be useful for you to update me on what's happening now. Then I'd like us to pick out your chief concerns – things that are a problem right now – and look at those in more detail. We can work together at seeing how we might improve the situation: standing back and taking stock often throws a new light on things. How does this sound to you?'

WORKING WITH INDIVIDUALS, OR WITH THE FAMILY AS A GROUP

The considerations noted earlier apply when deciding whether or not to include the patient in the stress-management programme. These include the needs of the relatives, e.g., would they feel inhibited by the presence of the patient? Do they need space and time to themselves to discuss issues?; as well as being realistic about what the patient can cope with: does the patient have the concentration and insight to participate in lengthy discussions about aspects of their own and their relatives' behaviour, and how these might be changed?

A flexible approach is required, allowing relatives at least some time to discuss difficulties without the patient present, but bringing the family together to assess situations or to plan change strategies that involve interactions between members. It is important to involve the relatives and patients in deciding how the sessions are organized, safeguarding that patients do not feel excluded. In cases where the husband or wife is the patient, we have most often found it advisable to include them for most of the work. Parallel sessions of assessment are often useful, where it is possible for two therapists to interview relative(s) and patient separately, without the patient feeling excluded.

Sometimes one family member tends to dominate the session. This can be because other members are reticent in giving their views, or because the dominant member 'answers for' the rest of the family – or usually a combination of both factors. In some cases, prompting quieter individuals to offer their opinion can be helpful, e.g., 'What do you do when this is happening?' 'How do you feel about that?', as well as giving a lot of feedback that you are listening and valuing the contributions they make, and making sure that anything you say is addressed to them as well as to the more verbal family members. It is important that you have been able to assess the less vocal member's particular problems and concerns, and that they are comfortable in facilitating any plans that require their involvement at home. It may sometimes be necessary to see them individually in order to establish that this is the case. These considerations and strategies apply whether it is the patient or another family member who contributes little to the joint sessions.

ASSESSMENT AND INTERVENTION FOR STRESS AND COPING PROBLEMS IN FAMILIES

The assessment steps are as follows. They may usually be completed in two sessions, with work on intervention strategies beginning in the second or third session, and thereafter continuing throughout the intervention either alone or in conjunction with patient goal-setting procedures (Chapter 7).

Session One

1. Explain nature and purpose of detailed questioning.
2. Give definition of stress.
3. Identify from interview and previous assessments a list of current stressors. Stressors here refer to patient-focused situations which the relative finds difficult to cope with, as well as stress responses associated with worrying thoughts, and also other themes of concern, which may or may not be patient-focused, e.g., finances, work, other family members.
4. Introduce self-monitoring of stressors.
5. Obtain details of resources available to the relative. Resources refers to strengths that the relative has which may be helpful to managing stress responses, e.g., social supports, work and leisure interests, success in managing other difficult situations. The latter will help to assess whether the relative needs to learn new skills, e.g., how to relax, how to be more assertive, or whether they have the skills but need help in implementing them. Much of this information should be available from the initial assessments.

Session Two

6. Review the self-monitoring and the list of stressors.
7. Target one or two specific situations and complete a detailed analysis, including the antecedents and consequences in terms of affects, cognitions, physical feelings, and behaviours, and the social context in which they occur.
8. Begin work on interventions on the basis of the analysis.

Session Three and Thereafter

9. Evaluate the outcomes of planned interventions, and modify where appropriate.
10. Generalize strategies to other situations.
11. Target further issues/situations for interventions.

Each of the components is described below, followed by some case examples.

Session One

1. Explain Nature and Purpose of Questioning

Following from the rationale, the purpose and format of further assessments should be explained, and the collaborative nature of this work
emphasized. This might be introduced as follows:

> I'd like us to spend some time talking about aspects of . . . problems
> that you find troublesome/find difficult to cope with/worry about
> particularly/are especially stressful. Trying to clearly identify the
> problems is the first step in working out solutions, and sometimes it
> helps just standing back and looking at situations in more detail. I'm
> particularly interested in any problems that are currently bothering
> you. These might be to do with . . . and his/her illness, or any other
> difficulties you are experiencing.

2. Stress

We have defined stress by using the transaction model: while some
events are stressful for everyone, each person has a unique response,
which to a greater or lesser extent may have some effect on the stressor
itself. Stress responses can be defined as any unpleasant or troublesome
thoughts, physical feelings, emotions, or behaviours. Examples, especially
those from the relatives' own experience, can be used to illustrate the
different modes of stress response, e.g., 'thoughts, such as you mentioned earlier about what will happen if she doesn't go back to college,
physical feelings, like the tension and palpitations you talked about;
emotions, such as anxiety or guilt or anger; and behaviours, such as the
argument you referred to when your son was lying on the settee.'

3. Identify form Interview and Previous Assessments a List of Current Stressors

Usually, the preliminary remarks about looking at problems and the
nature of stress will be sufficient prompts to facilitate discussion of difficulties. If the relatives are unclear about what is required, or are reticent
to talk, however, then information gathered from earlier assessments can
be used as prompts. Information sources are the RAI, the FQ, the GHQ,
and themes or specific situations which were identified in the education
sessions. For example, 'You mentioned in our earlier talk that you found
Jill's staying in bed bothered you. Is this still a problem at home?', or,
'I noticed on the form that you filled out [FQ] that John sometimes
doesn't answer when you speak to him, and you found that upsetting.
We talked a bit about that when I gave you the information about the
illness last week. Has that happened this week?' Or, more generally,
'When you filled out the form about your feelings, you indicated that you

sometimes felt panicky [had difficulty sleeping/were run down]. Could you tell me a bit more about that?' In the case of parental homes where the parents are interviewed conjointly, similarities and differences in terms of sources of concern might be highlighted.

The goal of the first session is principally to map out the triggers of stress responses and general themes of concern, although it is useful to begin to assess the contexts in which they occur, how the relative responds to them, and how the behaviour of other people, particularly the family, modify these responses. In the case of relatives of patients with longstanding illness, it is also useful to see how problems and coping responses have changed over time. For relatives who feel they have 'tried everything', it may be necessary to help them to reappraise their coping responses, to emphasize that coping is multifaceted, and to thus persuade them that all possible modifications to their behaviour have not been exhausted; or that a consensus in coping among family members may be as important as the efforts of individual members. The therapist should obtain feedback from the relatives about these themes, and be alert to the relatives' feeling that their previous efforts are being criticized.

The stressful triggers and themes of concern may include:

1. Patient behaviours, such as given in the earlier examples.
2. Disagreements between family members about how aspects of the illness should be interpreted and managed at home.
3. Concerns or worries about real or hypothetical situations to do with the illness, e.g., what will other people think of her? What if he doesn't take the medication/She gets ill again/He loses his job/?
4. Concerns or worries about life problems that are not specifically patient-focused, e.g., problems associated with the relative's other children, difficulties at work, financial problems.

4. Introduce Self-Monitoring of Stressors

Self-monitoring is an effective way of both collecting more reliable information about relatives' well-being in their day-to-day lives, and of educating relatives about the nature of their stress responses: when they occur, what triggers them, and how they react in terms of their affects, feelings, and behaviours.

The monitoring we have used asks relatives to note down on prepared forms (Table 6.1) instances when they feel 'stressed' or when problems occur. The first example asks the relative to record on a daily basis situations which were associated with stress responses or problems, and gives a reminder definition of what is meant by stress. The second asks the relative to record not only the situation or context in which the stress

Table 6.1 Examples of Self-Monitoring Forms for Relatives to Record Problems and Stressful Situations at Home

1. Please note down situations when you felt stressed or where problems occurred at home.				
Day/Date	**Situation** (what was happening, where, who was there)		**Feelings** (Stressed, unpleasant or troublesome thoughts, emotions behaviour or physical feelings)	

2. Please note down situations when you felt stressed or where problems occurred at home.				
Day/Date	**Situation**	**How did you feel?**	**What did you think?**	**What did you do?**

response occurred, but the consequences and details of the nature of the stress response in terms of thoughts, feelings, and behaviour.

The complexity of the recording will depend on factors such as the ease or difficulty with which the relative fills in forms, as well as how they perceive the value of monitoring and recording. Both of these factors may be modified to some extent by the therapist, the first by giving guided practice of completion before the relatives attempt to fill out forms at home, and the second by emphasizing the benefits of the monitoring, and paying attention to its completion in the sessions. In reality, by sticking to the level of monitoring the relative is comfortable with, there is a good chance they will reliably complete. This may mean simplifying the forms, e.g., devizing a checklist whereby the relative need tick only the occurrence/absence of specified situations. However, simpler recording will mean more work has to be done with the relative in sessions, working out the details of situations retrospectively. Where relatives fail to complete even the simplest forms between sessions, it is best to accept this rather than to insist they keep trying. One can ask the relatives to make a mental note of situations and their responses, and spend some of the session completing retrospective recordings with them.

Before the relative completes the form as a 'homework' assignment, it should be tried out during the session, using examples the relative has given from the preceding week. Where there is more than one relative involved, e.g., a parental household or with participating siblings, individuals should be encouraged to complete their records independently, although communication of records need not be discouraged. When the patient is participating, it is important to include them as a participant in the recording to reduce any feelings that they are being 'observed', particularly in the case of patients with persecutory ideas. They may be offered the same opportunity to record stressors, but it is advisable to check how they feel about this, and to assess whether it is a realistic task for them to perform, given concentration difficulties or other constraints.

5. Obtain Details of Resources Available to the Relative

A number of resource areas need to be considered, since they will be important when selecting intervention strategies. Much of this information will be available from initial assessments, for example, interests and recreational activities that may be used to distract the relative from worrying thoughts; friends who may be useful in assisting them to recommence activities outside the home, or to assist them with problem-solving, particularly when the relative alone with the patient. It may be necessary to find out what the relative used to enjoy doing and who they used to see, since interests and social relationships may have been given up because of problems with the illness.

Session Two

6. Review the Self-Monitoring and the List of Stressors

The second session should ideally take place within about a week. The therapist reviews the list of stressors compiled at the previous session, and examines the record sheet with the relative(s). Did the relative find the issues they had previously discussed caused any concern during the week? 'When we last met, we talked about the situations and concerns that were troubling you, and we made a list of the these things [briefly summarize]. We also talked about stress and how it affects us. You were going to try and note down details of situations and your responses during the week. Did you manage to do this?'

7. and 8. Target One or Two Specific Situations
and Complete a Detailed Analysis, Leading to intervention Strategies

Once the broad problem areas have been defined, a careful description of specific situations is sought. Where relatives have completed self-monitoring records, these can be used to begin a more detailed analysis of the situations occurring at home. Otherwise, it is best to look at situations that have occurred recently, preferably in the last week, so that recall problems are reduced.

The behavioural analysis seeks to build up a detailed picture of exactly what was happening before the problem situation began. It is useful to ask the relative to give a picture of the day's events in general terms, and then to describe in more detail what preceded the key event:

1. What happens in the specific situation; who is present, what they are doing.
2. What the relative is doing (including their thoughts, feelings, and behaviour) before, during, and after the key events.
3. What are the behaviours of the patient, family members, or other people before, during, and after key events, and how they effect the stress responses of the relative.
4. What were the outcomes for all concerned.

The function of the analysis is to pinpoint the problems and to explore with the relative(s) the factors which are precipitating and maintaining their distress in this particular set of events, how similar/dissimilar this is to other situations, and what makes things better or worse. Having examined the sequence of events (including the relative's thoughts and feelings) which result in the relative feeling distressed, realistic ways to intervene to reduce the problems can be explored in collaboration with the relatives. This clarification of events *per se* is sometimes sufficient to permit relatives to reappraise the problem and suggest alternatives. Some general guidelines in analyzing situations include:

1. Break global problems down into constituent problems.
2. Where the precipitants of stress responses are patient-focused, consider whether it is possible to involve the patient in change strategies, for example, using problem-solving or goal-setting (Chapter 7), or a non-family-based intervention, such as medication change or day-care placement, or whether it is more realisitic/appropriate to focus on changing the relative's response, or where a combination of efforts seems feasible.
3. Consider which aspects of the relative's behaviours, thoughts, and physical feelings are contributing to the problem.

These guidelines are best illustrated by the case examples that begin on page 100 before general principles and techniques of stress management with the family are discussed.

9. Evaluate the Outcomes Modify Where Appropriate

It is important to set the evaluation of proposed interventions high on the agenda for the next session. If the relative complies with record-keeping, then some form of continuous monitoring of outcomes can be kept. Target variables to be recorded might include the relative's subjective feelings, for example, distress, anxiety, anger; or their perceived ability to cope with a situation; or some aspect of the patient's behaviour which the intervention has targeted for change, for example, frequency or intensity of anger outbursts; time of getting up; time spent in the house alone. Efforts to implement the rehearsed plans should be reinforced, and improvements on target variables can be charted or graphed and shown to the relative. A careful analysis of any difficulties and feedback from the relative on how they felt about the plan's implementation are important. Possible problems include:

Plan Not Implemented
Sometimes this may be a case of 'the problem just didn't arise', or 'the problem's no longer an issue'. In such cases it is important to try to establish why the problem has not arisen/is not an issue when it did/was previously. Common answers include: the patient behaviour has not changed, but the relative has reappraised the behaviour and is no longer concerned by it; the behaviour/situation is not occurring with the same frequency – possibly the relative was mistaken about the frequency, or the relative is no longer bothered by it and therefore less vigilant for its occurrence; a new problem now preoccupies the relative, so old concerns have become fairly insignificant.

It is worthwhile discussing with the relatives the reasons for the problem or their perceptions of the problem changing. In some cases the relative might be persuaded to implement the plan even though it is no longer a priority concern, because it might become an issue at a later date. Sometimes there are issues of validity of problems to discuss: relatives may feel they have been overly preoccupied with what others might consider 'trivial' problems; or they may have difficulty coming to terms with accepting help, and wish to give the impression they can cope. As always, it is best to accept the relative's viewpoint, and to let them know that you consider people who live with the problems of schizophrenia very good at coping, but that the illness presents exceptional demands. A number of small problems can add up to a large difficulty, and talking issues over with people outside the family situation can sometimes be helpful.

Plan Did Not Work
A careful description of exactly what the relatives did in response to the targeted situation is necessary, and further rehearsal or modifications will be required. Possibly the plan was partially successful, and the positive gains need to be emphasized so the relative is encouraged to continue. This is particularly true with relatives who are significantly depressed, or where morale is low after years of attempting to cope while seeing little or no improvement in the patient.

10. Generalize Strategies to Other Situations

The therapist should attempt to assist the relatives to draw general conclusions or common themes about the efficacy of particular techniques in specific situations, for example, 'Do you think we can use the success you had in coping with temper outbursts in other situations?', or, 'What do you think were the reasons for your success in coping with John's temper outbursts? How can we use these in other situations?' Planning for the maintenance of successful strategies can also be important. Sometimes relatives commence plans with enthusiasm but later discontinue, perhaps because a perceived crisis is over, or because other problems divert their attention. Continued monitoring of planned interventions and outcomes as noted above is one way of checking maintenance. If the therapist reinforces the continued efforts of the relative and discusses changes and problems, they are more likely to persevere with new coping techniques.

Case examples follow. The first two examples were cited earlier in this chapter.

Example 1

The patient is a 38-year-old man, John, whose behaviour has been extremely disturbed for the past 18 years. Although there are periods of improvement, and the nature of his fears change over time, he has continued to have persecutory delusions and auditory hallucinations. He lives alone with his elderly mother, Mary, who is socially isolated. There are no other relatives locally, and the mother is financially restricted and has health and mobility problems. His mother highlights her son's tirades against imagined persecutors, currently policemen, social security officials, and health workers, as the source of much of her fear and anxiety.

Mary described herself as feeling 'continually on edge' at home, and welcomed the opportunity to discuss her feelings. The RAI and the education sessions had indicated that she felt guilty about her son's situation, and queried her own role in 'making him ill'. The onset of his illness was shortly after the sudden death of her husband and their temporary move to the south of England, and she was concerned that these events had caused his illness.

Mary had had little direct contact with hospital or community health services, and felt that she and John were a nuisance. She interpreted various comments from medical staff over the years as suggesting that she made John worse. These were references to her 'overprotective behaviour': John did no housework or cooking and refused to attend the day-centre. Mary looked after his personal needs and was rarely separated from him.

In the past John had made two suicide attempts. He had broken windows and kicked down doors in the house, but it was several years since he had been physically destructive, and there was no history of violence to his mother or to anyone else. Mary felt that his disturbed behaviour reflected on her: current examples of such behaviour were accusing neighbours of spying on him; leaving the room when visitors came; shouting at officials at the social security office and the local health centre.

Mary's GHQ score was high on all subscales, and on the FQ she reported that the felt unable to control a lot of his problem behaviours. She had no close friends. Her other two children did not live locally, and she saw them rarely. Although there were no pressing financial difficulties, she had only a small pension. She was 70 and had a history of angina and arthritis.

John declined to participate in sessions with the therapists, and was at first suspicious that they were sent by the social security office to check whether he was fit for work and thus not entitled to social security benefits. However, simple and repeated reassurance seemed to calm these fears. Throughout the work with his mother he would phone the therapists and seek further reassurance, and latterly would also seek reassurance about persecutory ideas. A simple statement that we/the police/the community nurse/ etc. were not trying to harm him/ take his benefits away/kill him was sufficient, followed by engaging him on another topic of conversation. From the outset we explained that we wanted to help his mother to understand his illness and to cope with her stress, and this explanation of involvment was acceptable to him.

At the first session, Mary had readily adopted the rationale for discussion her feelings. As noted earlier, she reported high levels of distress. She repeated some of the problems that had been apparent in the RAI, and the list of current problems was as follows: fears that John would be destructive in the house; being woken in the night by him getting up, and lying awake worrying about what he might be doing; worries about what would happen to him if she was ill or died; concern about the neighbours when John shouted at them or knocked on the wall; distress when he started accusatory talk about officials.

She reported that in the past she had tended to spend more time dissuading him of his ideas than she now did, and she felt that as a consequence he got less angry at home. She also said she tried not to let him see that she was upset, and tried to keep it to herself.

At the second session, Mary had completed the record sheet (Table 6.2) and had noted down daily instances of feeling upset. Most of the situations concerning John's behaviour had been precipitated either by specific events or by thoughts. The majority of the situations fell into the categories described above. Since the problem was very much Mary's mind, the first situation that was analyzed in more detail was John's behaviour the day before his monthly modecate injection, when he annouced to his mother his intention of phoning the health centre

Table 6.2   Case Example 1: Self-Monitoring Form
Please note down situations when you felt stressed or where problems occurred at home.

Day	Situation	How did you feel?	What did you think?	What did you do?
Thurs night	Heard J walking about downstairs.	Tense.	What's he doing? Why can't he sleep?	Lay awake worrying.
Fri morn	J complained that a TV character was getting at him.	A bit annoyed.	I'll have to switch off TV.	Switched off TV.
Sat	Social security payment didn't arrive. J upset & said people were on to him.	Tense.	Here we go again. He'll be on about this all day.	Tried to keep out of J's way.
Mon	Next door neighbour called in. J went to his room & wouldn't come out for hours.	Tense & worried.	I can't see anybody without J getting upset.	Tried to persuade J to come out of his room.
Tues	J said he was going to phone the health centre & say he wasn't having the injection.	Tense, upset.	What will people think? What if he doesn't get his injection?	Tried to persuade J not to phone. Argued.
Tues night	Lying in bed.	Couldn't sleep.	What will become of us both.	Lay awake.

and telling them what he thought of them: to verbally abuse them and tell them that he wasn't going to have his injection because they were only trying to make him ill. Mary recorded that she had felt tense and upset. She had attempted to reason with John not to phone and there had been arguments, with John shouting and swearing at his mother. This situation had continued throughout the day, with John threatening to phone, and Mary repeatedly attempting to dissuade him. Eventually he had phoned and verbally abused the community nurse.

From the mother's record and further questioning, the analysis was as follows:

The mother was asked when she first began to feel stressed. She reported that she picked up 'signs' that John was 'going to be difficult' some time before the problem began. These signs were 'a look in his eyes', not saying as much as usual, and getting up earlier than usual. Additionally, it emerged that the scenario of threatening to phone the health centre around the time of his injection was a regular occurrence, and Mary agreed that she was probably anticipating trouble and more vigilant of John's behaviour.

In response to her anticipating and John's behaviour, Mary felt tense and had physical anxiety symptoms. This tension heightened when John began to talk about the health centre, and thoughts such as 'What will I do if he misses his injection and gets more ill?' and, 'What will they think of me, letting him phone up and make a nuisance of himself?' had passed through her mind. These thoughts appeared to be important to maintaining her distress. At first she tried to distract herself with housework, but after half an hour or so of John going on, she had started to attempt to reason with him, then to dissuade him from phoning, and arguments had ensured. At about three in the afternoon, he had phoned, told the community nurse that he 'bloody well wasn't having the needle', and that 'he knew why he was ill, it was those chemicals they kept forcing him to have'. Mary had felt angry and ashamed, and remained feeling tense and upset for the rest of the day. The nurse had tried to persuade John to come in for his injection and he did so, not the following day when it was due, but some three days later.

This situation was compared with other times when John was due for his injection. The pattern was similar, with Mary getting upset to a greater or lesser extent on different occasions. The outcome – that John did eventually go for his injection within a few days of it being due – was consistent across situations.

THE INTERVENTION

It was noted earlier that an intervention directed at reducing the mother's anxiety response was felt to be most appropriate in this situation. Role-play was used to help elicit her behaviour and thoughts in the situation, with the therapist taking the part of the son. Alternative strategies were role-played, including the situation where the mother took a more confrontative dissuasive role, arguing against her son's beliefs and urging him to get the injection. This approach was rejected by the mother, who had earlier reported that the more she challenged his beliefs the more difficult John's behaviour became, and this theory was endorsed by the therapist. A lower-key approach was discussed, and role-played, which involved the mother telling John that it was important to get his injection, but to phone the centre if he wanted to speak to the staff about it. Four or five repetitions were necessary before the mother felt comfortable with this approach. In the first attempt the mother's tone was abrupt, and the roles were reversed, with the therapist modelling the mother to facilitate her understanding of the importance of her tone of voice. The consequences of such a strategy were discussed.

The mother also felt responsible for the son's behaviour, and that by 'letting him get on with it' people would think badly of her: 'the staff will think I'm terrible for letting him speak like that, causing them all that trouble', and, 'if I don't try and persuade him he may not get his medication'. These ideas were challenged, principally along the lines that, firstly, her son had a severe mental illness of which his delusional beliefs were a symptom and she was not reponsible for his behaviour; secondly, the staff were trained and employed specifically to help people like John; thirdly, he invariably did get his medication.

Work was also done helping the mother to calm her anticipatory anxiety when she expected the situation to arise, chiefly through the rehearsal of positive self statements, such as, 'I have gone over how to handle this calmly with the therapist. Nothing terrible will happen by letting him phone up the health centre if that's what he feels like doing.' When the mother felt confident, the strategies were implemented at home. Initially the mother still felt tense, but gained confidence that her new approach was successful: she reported less haranguing from the son. She was encouraged to persevere, and although her son continued to complain and phone the centre every month, she felt he was less angry, and she felt much less distressed by the situation.

The principal components of the intervention were:

1. Reappraising the consequences of her son's behaviour.
2. Reappaising her own role in her son's behaviour.
3. Challenging beliefs about what others thought of her.
4. Teaching anxiety control through positive self-statements.
5. Changing her behavioural response to reduce the challenging of the son's beliefs and subsequent arguments.

Work was done on encouraging the mother to generalize the approaches to other difficult situations. For example, there were many parallels between the medication-refusal situation described and the mother's concern for John's delusional talk about the neighbours. In both cases, central to the mother's distress were fears of what people thought about her, and unrealistic beliefs that she could control John's behaviour. She was also helped to address her needs through goal-setting for building up her interests, activities, and social contacts outside of the home and her son's problems.

Example 2

The patient, Andrew, is a 30-year-old man who lives with his parents and a younger sibling. He has had three acute episodes of schizophrenia, and is currently free of positive symptoms, but does little at home, spending long periods lying on the bed. His father gets very angry about his lack of activity, and there are family disagreements triggered by the issue.

The family members were in agreement that they were willing to try anything that might assist Andrew. The father reported being increasingly worried by his son's lack of progress and the fact that Andrew had not had a job since the illness began three years earlier, and that he had few friends. He had tried to engage the son's interest in a number of activities without lasting success, but felt strongly that his son needed to do more, and that lying around the house was partly responsible for his problems. The mother was more overtly distressed, as was evident from the GHQ responses and her reports of disturbed sleep and time off work during the son's last breakdown. She felt the family had to accept that Andrew was severely handicapped by his illness, and that making demands on him was likely to bring on further acute episodes. The younger son had little knowledge about the illness, but felt somewhat resentful at the problems it had led to in the family. He had attended the education sessions and reported having a better understanding of Andrew's difficulties. All the family except Andrew were in full-time employment.

Andrew was very co-operative with the therapists and had insight into the nature of this illness. At the time of the intervention he was free from positive symptoms, but was mildly depressed. He did not get on well with his younger brother and they frequently argued, but felt that his parents were supportive. He reported feeling bored at home, but did not know what to do outside the house, and had lost touch with most of his friends, and felt lacking in energy.

The first stress-management session was attended by the parents only, although the nature of the session was described to Andrew. It was felt that the parents would feel less inhibited in expressing their concerns if Andrew was not present, and he was in agreement. The younger brother was unable to attend the sessions, and the family agreed to discuss the content with him at home, which was also acceptable to Andrew.

The mother emphasized that although she often felt upset by the effects of the illness on Andrew, she was careful not to display her concerns. The therapist attempted to give positive feedback to this approach, while focusing on how she might benefit from sharing her concerns, and that keeping them to oneself is often hard to cope with, especially over long periods. The situations that concerned the mother were reported as general worries rather than specific situations. These were: whether Andrew would continue to take his medication (he had a history of medication non-compliance); the fear that he would be acutely ill again, and if so that he might not recover; concern that the younger son was argumentative with Andrew and threatened to leave home. The father said he tended to get 'worked up' about Andrew's lack of activity, but that this was not a current issue since Andrew was now attending day-care. The mother's concern over medication was used to illustrate the components of anxiety responses and how these might be recorded, and it was suggested that both parents attempt to note down instances on the record sheets at home.

At the second session, the records were reviewed. The mother's recording was more comprehensive than the father's, showing a number of situations which had triggered anxiety over the week. In particular there had been an argument between her and her husband about Andrew's untidiness, which was analyzed during the session.

The argument had occurred on a weekday morning when the parents were getting ready to go out to work. The father had complained that Andrew had left the bathroom in a mess. The mother had said she could not see how this concerned him so much, since it was her who always cleaned the bathroom, and for that matter he might spend a bit more time helping with the housework himself. The father had then got annoyed with his wife, and had said that part of Andrew's problem was that he spent too much time doing nothing, and that his wife was too soft with the boy. Eventually the couple left for work. The mother reported that she had felt upset throughout the day, and that there had been an atmosphere between them for several following days, although the issue had not been further discussed or resolved.

From the mother's record and further questioning of both parents, the analysis of the problem was as follows:

The mother said she had felt rushed getting ready that morning and that she was preoccupied with a number of tasks when the argument began. She had felt angry that her husband had started to go on about Andrew, mainly because she felt she was the one who was worried about him and spent time trying to talk to him and find ways of occupying his time; she felt that nagging him was not the solution, and had queried her husband's lack of feeling for his son's problems. Thoughts such as these had concerned her for some time after the argument.

The father's recall of the incident was questioned. Could he remember what had bothered him that morning? He suggested that he had probably been feeling in a bad mood that day, and that although his son's untidiness had irritated him that morning, 'nine times out of ten, I wouldn't have said anything'. 'When asked what he was feeling bad about?', it emerged that he had some problems at work, and had not felt able to discuss these with his wife because he knew she was preoccupied with concerns about Andrew and did not want to worry her further. He felt that most of the conversation for the past few months had revolved around Andrew and his problems. He was also concerned that the younger son was not getting much attention.

The situation described was broken down into two difficulties and presented back to the parents: 'There seem to be two issues here. One is how to respond to Andrew's untidiness, in his case in the bathroom, but I think you've mentioned other aspects of his not helping in the house. It would be best if you could both agree on how this is best dealt with. And secondly, how Andrew's problems have meant that you have had less time to to talk to each other about the things that concern you. Does this briefly summarize the issues?'

THE INTERVENTION

Although patient-focused behaviour was the trigger for feelings of stress in this situation, it was apparent that communication issues between the parents were also contributing to the cause and maintenance of stress responses. Breaking the problem down into two components which were acceptable to the relatives helped to reduce the size of the overall problem and to make it more manageable. The concrete problem of how to deal with the untidiness was targeted first; we have found relatives often feel more comfortable discussing patient-focused problems than in analyzing other relationships, and the former is an entry into the latter.

Since Andrew was willing and able to contribute to resolving difficulties, it was felt important to include him in this aspect of the intervention. The parents were encouraged to talk to him about leaving the bathroom in a mess, which was rehearsed during the sessions with the therapist. It emerged that both the father's and mother's beliefs about the illness needed to be dealt with if a common policy were to be successful. The father's idea was just to tell Andrew, 'I think you should start tidying up after yourself.' The mother felt this was too critical, and that Andrew might not be able to remember or have the energy to do it.

The parents were reminded about negative symptoms, and that prompts and reminders were often useful in facilitating behaviour, especially if these were offered in a non-critical manner. The father had difficulty rehearsing such a strategy, believing that, 'I shouldn't have to remind him to do ordinary things.' The mother felt, 'He's ill, so why are we making such an issue over a bit of a mess in the bathroom?' The father's ideas were dealt with by further discussion of negative symptoms; the mother's by pointing out that resolving this untidiness might help

Andrew in other ways: he had formerly been interested in his appearance and in taking care of his clothes, and had expressed an interest in co-operating, and this small change might help facilitate change in other more important things.

The agreed plan was that the parents would discuss the untidiness with Andrew, acknowledging that people with his illness often find ordinary things more of an effort than they used to. They said they would remind him to tidy the bathroom after himself, and/or would help him to do so. This was acceptable to Andrew. The parents were encouraged to challenge beliefs contrary to this plan as outlined above, and to inform the younger brother of the strategies. They decided they would also request that the younger brother tidied the bathroom after himself, and he agreed this was reasonable.

Problem-solving was used to facilitate the parents having more time for each other. They decided to revive the habit of going for a meal once a week.

It was reported that Andrew became tidier in the bathroom. The mother used prompts successfully, while the father reported he felt it was less of an issue to him, and that since talking the matter through he no longer felt irritated. The parents occasionally went out for meals, although not once a week. They decided that discussions about Andrew should not take place during the morning rush before work.

The parents were encouraged to generalize the strategies to other situations.

The principal components of the intervention were:

1. Encouraging the parents to have a consensus strategy for the problem.
2. Facilitating discussion of the problem between the parents and the son.
3. Reappaising the son's behaviour and challenging the parents' beliefs.
4. Using alternative beliefs as self-statements to calm feelings of stress.
5. Teaching the use of prompts to initiate patient behaviours.
6. Using problem-solving to enable the parents to have more time together.

Example 3

Mrs Smith is 53 and has a 20-year history of schizophrenia, with frequent hospitalizations over that period. She continues to experience some auditory hallucinations and delusions of a paranoid nature, but copes with them reasonably well, principally through withdrawal. At home there is little behavioural disturbance, and she copes with housework and shopping, but she sleeps a lot and goes out infre-quently. She lives with her husband who is unemployed but who works voluntarily for a political party several hours a day. The couple manage financially on a very restricted budget. They have two children who are married and do not live locally.

The RAI and questionnaire assessments indicated that Mr Smith experienced considerable tension, which was precipitated by his wife's accusatory outbursts when she was acutely ill, and to a lesser extent by her inactivity. At the first session, the couple were seen together since Mrs Smith said she would feel uncomfortable if she felt that people were talking about her. Mrs Smith was able to disclose some of the situations which made her feel 'agitated' and 'tired'. Principally these involved going out of the house, and money issues. Mr Smith said that he was not stressed now that his wife's behaviour was calmer, and felt that it was his wife and not him who needed help with tension at present.

The therapist did not attempt to directly dissuade Mr Smith from this viewpoint, but focused on if and how he was aware that his wife was agitated, before asking how such behaviour affected him. In the context of this questioning, Mr Smith described recognizing that his wife was tense when she left the room, and that he felt concern and sometimes irritation when this happened. Mrs Smith was similarly asked how she was able to tell if her husband was agitated. She had difficulty pinpointing situations, but felt he sometimes got annoyed with her. Both partners were asked to keep a record of their feelings during the week: Mrs Smith was asked to record her agitation and tiredness; and Mr Smith to record his concern and irritation.

At the next session, Mrs Smith said she had been unable to keep the record, but Mr Smith had completed his record form daily. There were four instances of him feeling irritated during the week, and on two occasions these feelings had occurred in the early evenings. In one example, the couple had been watching TV when Mrs Smith had left the room abruptly. Mr Smith had gone to look for his wife, and had found her lying on the bed. He had continued to watch TV alone for the rest of the evening, but had felt annoyed. This situation was analyzed in detail during the session.

Mr Smith was encouraged to describe the situation of watching the TV together in more detail. Although he had a preference for watching current event and discussion programmes, they had been watching a comedy, Mrs Smith's preferred programme that evening. According to Mr Smith, his wife's exit from the lounge was 'out of the blue'. At first he thought she had just gone to the toilet or had gone to do something in the kitchen, but after five minutes and she did not return, he had begun to feel annoyed:

'What thoughts went through your head?'

'I thought how the evening had been spoiled yet again. I felt she was deliberately avoiding being with me. It's difficult when you spend so much time in the house together and there's no conversation. I'd thought that evening we could at least watch the telly together, especially when she'd picked the programme. I might as well have gone out for the night.'

'What did you do?'

'I tried to watch the programme, but I kept wondering what she was doing and feeling annoyed. Eventually I went upstairs and found her lying on the bed. That annoyed me, but I didn't say anything, since I know that arguing doesn't do her any good. I just left her to it.'

'How long did you continue to feel annoyed?'

'The rest of the evening. I decided that in future I might as well watch the programmes that I was interested in, or go out to the club.'

It emerged that the situation had not been discussed with Mrs Smith, but that she had felt that Mr Smith was annoyed. 'You can tell by the way he slams the doors and doesn't say anything.' She was able to recall the evening, and was asked to describe how she had felt when she left the room. Mrs Smith reported that she found watching television difficult, and the particular characters in the comedy had made her feel 'peculiar', 'as if they were getting at me', although she was unable to specify why. She had left the room to get away from the feelings and thoughts, and had gone to bed since this usually made her feel better. Her husband's coming to find her, and her inference that he was annoyed had made her feel agitated so she had continued to lie down, and had eventually gone to sleep.

The situation was reviewed by the therapist: 'What seems to be happening is that Iris is sometimes disturbed by watching the television, and this happened on the evening we have talked about. She finds getting away from the TV and lying down a good way to cope with these feelings. However, Brian, you would like to spend more time with Iris, and you felt that your efforts to do so were met with rejection and this made you feel annoyed. Perhaps we could sort out a plan for dealing with this kind of situation which takes into account both your points of view. How does this sound to you?'

THE INTERVENTION

Mrs Smith said that it was difficult for her to know when she was likely to get upset by the TV; sometimes there was no problem watching it, while other times she just felt the need to get away. She did not feel able to explain why, since this could lead to having to talk about her feelings, which made her feel worse. Mr Smith said he found his wife's behaviour difficult to rationalize when it occurred at home, although it would seem to be part of her illness, and that lying down was her way of coping.

It was agreed that if Mrs Smith felt the need to withdraw to the bedroom while watching TV or doing anything else while her husband was at home, she should try and let him know by saying she was feeling unwell. Mr Smith was encouraged to rehearse coping statements that did not personalize her behaviour against him, such as, 'Iris is going to lie down because she feels unwell', and to distract himself with other activities if he felt himself becoming irritated. A number of these were brainstormed with the help of his wife, including phoning a friend or his daughter; watching a current affairs programme, or reading a book or newspaper, or going for a walk or for a drink at the club. It was agreed that he would check to see how his wife was and suggest she might like to come back to the lounge, but that he should not press the point.

These strategies were rehearsed during the session, using the reported incident of Mrs Smith's abrupt departure from watching the TV as an example. Some difficulties included Mr Smith wanting to find out just what it was that made his wife feel uncomfortable with the programme, and his wife's reluctance to disclose her feelings; and some abruptness in his manner of enquiring whether she would like to return to the lounge. When the situation had been rehearsed several times, the couple were encouraged to try it out at home.

The strategies were partially successful, in that Mrs Smith had been able to mention her withdrawal before going up to the bedroom, and Mr Smith had felt less annoyed through reappraising her behaviour as illness feelings, but he had later tried to persuade her that she would be better to get up. His persuasions were unsuccessful, and triggered more feelings of annoyance on his part, and an increased need to withdraw on Mrs Smith's part. It was decided that Mr Smith should simply leave his wife to decide whether and when to return downstairs, and his feelings about this were discussed. Mr Smith was concerned this might lead to his wife taking to her bed more and more as she had done for periods during her illness, but he agreed to try out the strategy. The frequency and duration of his wife's withdrawals decreased.

The principal components of the intervention were:

1. Facilitating a shared analysis of the problem.
2. Helping the husband to reappraise his wife's behaviour and to challenge his beliefs.
3. Using self-statements and distraction to reduce irritation.
4. Changing the husband's behavioural response to his wife's withdrawal.

Mr Smith was able to generalize some of the strategies to other situations. For example, he reported feeling less irritated when his wife did not answer when he spoke to her. He was able to attribute this behaviour to some preoccupation connected with her illness, rather than to personalize it as a deliberate snub or disinterest in what he had to say, and found that if he left his remarks to a time when she seemed less preoccupied with her thoughts, he usually got an answer. Later, problem-solving was used to increase the couple's shared activities.

GENERAL PRINCIPLES OF STRESS-MANAGEMENT INTERVENTIONS

We hope the case examples have clarified some of the assessment and intervention procedures described earlier, as well as highlighting both the variation and common themes in working with families to reduce stress. Some of the general principles of the work can be summarized as follows:

1. Where some stress responses are triggered by patient-focused events, it is best to begin work with concrete examples rather than to first tackle more general themes of concern (e.g., worries about hypothetical situations associated with the illness, such as, 'what if he gets ill again'/'he doesn't take medication'/'something happens to me'). The value of first focusing on concrete situations is that specific interventions can be tried out and reviewed, and the relatives get immediate feedback from implementing alternative strategies. Also, success in dealing with specific situations can reduce some of the general worries and anticipatory anxieties about possible future events.
2. It is important to invest time in a detailed analysis of problem situations, many of which arise from cumulative difficulties and tensions. Their context needs to be understood if interventions are to be effective.
3. Role plays of the situations are often useful in facilitating an assessment and in planning behaviour changes, where targeted situations involve interactions between family members.
4. It is important that all details of strategies for change have been covered before the plan is implemented. General advice such as, 'It's best not to argue'; 'Try and distract yourself'; 'Try talking to him about it'; or 'Don't get upset' can be unhelpful for the relative, who may rightly respond 'That's easier said than done!', and either not implement the advice, or try to implement but fail because they are unsure of what to do or say, or because there are unforseen consequences to their actions.
5. It is important to be alert to 'cognitive blocks', which relatives may have to changing their behaviours. In the second example, the father's belief that prompting his son to perform everyday tasks was unnecessary is one of the most common of such blocks in relatives changing their strategies for dealing with negative symptoms; in the

first example the belief that others would criticize the mother for the son's behaviour was a strong determinant in her persevering with unsuccessful attempts to dissuade her son from acting on his delusions.

6. Although patient-focused situations may be the focus of stress responses, in families with multiple members it is often the real or perceived reactions of other relatives that trigger and maintain stress responses. Common problems here are disagreements about the management and understanding of patient behaviours, and dissatisfactions about the amount of time family members invest, or fail to invest, in helping the patient, while neglecting the concerns of other members of the family. Discussion of problems, as noted below, will help to resolve such disagreements.

7. In helping the relatives to change their coping responses, the therapist should be guided by the themes of EE assessment. Attempts to control, limit, or change patient behaviours through repeated verbal persuasion, threats, or arguments are usually ineffective and may cause the relatives and patient considerable distress; similarly, attempts to ameliorate problems by doing everything for the patient, and becoming a buffer between him or her and the outside world are not only ineffective in the long term, but are likely to have an adverse effect on the relatives' well-being.

COPING STRATEGIES AND STRESS REDUCTION TECHNIQUES

We have repeatedly cautioned against work with families being seen as the application of a set of techniques, and emphasized the need for interventions to be tailored to the individual problems families present. Within the framework of individual analysis, however, there are a number of intervention strategies that are common to many interventions, most of which were illustrated in the case examples in this chapter. Chapter 7 concentrates on problem-based coping; here we are concerned with strategies that aim to directly decrease relatives' distress.

Problem Discussion and Analysis

The shared discussion and analysis of problem situations is not only necessary for finding solutions and alternative ways of coping, but can be sufficient for relatives to resolve situations (Falloon *et al.*, 1984). One of the functions of discussions about problems between family members is to facilitate a shared understanding of how each person perceives the problem. For example, in the third case example (page 108) the wife's need to withdraw from the TV was her way of coping with her symptoms, whereas for her husband it seemed to be a deliberate means of avoiding being with him. Sometimes the correction of misinterpretations about the behaviour of another family member resolves the problem, or at least permits the family to generate appropriate solutions and reach a consensus on how it is best resolved.

The importance of the timing and location of discussions needs to be understood if relatives are to use discussion-based problem-solving at home. Often, people only 'discuss' problems at the height of a crisis, or when they are feeling angry and tense. The so-called discussion rapidly becomes an argument, which is then used as a reason why talking about problems with family members is not helpful. It may be necessary to help relatives to sort out the best times for talking about difficulties; when none of the parties is likely to feel tired, tense, or too busy.

Frequently, there may be only one relative residing with the patient, and the relative does not have a confidante with whom to discuss problems; or for various reasons the relative feels disinclined to talk to others about the situation at home due to a fear of seeming disloyal to the patient, embarrassment about mental illness problems, or a dislike of letting others know they have problems. Building a social-support network, including people with whom the relative feels comfortable to discuss difficulties, may be an important goal of the intervention, particularly when the patient's behaviour is severely disturbed. Often local groups of the National Schizophrenia Fellowship can provide some support.

Modifying the Beliefs of Relatives

The way in which the relative perceives and interprets the behaviour of the patient, and other family members, often contributes to their emotional and behavioural responses. Some common 'thinking errors' which can lead to distress or management problems include the following:

Misinterpretations or Faulty Attributions About Behaviours

Positive and negative symptom-related behaviours, such as delusional talk, failure to respond when spoken to, inappropriate giggling and affect, social withdrawal, and underactivity, may be perceived to be controllable by the patient, or by the relative. Examples of how such thinking can give rise to upset or annoyance were given in the case studies: the husband who personalized his wife's withdrawal and thought she was deliberately avoiding him (page 108); the mother who thought she should be able to stop her son's persecutory ideas and behaviour, which she believed were offensive to health care staff (page 100).

Unrealistic or Uncertain Expectations

Beliefs that the patient should be doing more; or have less problems; or uncertainty about what the family should realistically expect of the patient are sources of concern for relatives. For example, in the example where the parents were unsure how much of the son's untidiness was symptom related (page 104).

Many of the thinking errors or negative thoughts that have been described by cognitive therapists in depressed or anxious people are evidenced in the thinking of distressed relatives: catastrophizing situations; taking responsibility for the patient's behaviour; jumping to conclusions; over-generalizing.

Sometimes, shared discussion and analysis of problem situations may be sufficient to rectify misinterpretations and other faulty assumptions about situations and behaviours of family members, or the education component may resolve unhelpful beliefs. However, in some cases further interventions may be necessary.

As with cognitive-behavioural interventions for people with other emotional problems (Hawton *et al.*, 1989), such unhelpful beliefs can be changed through a combination of discussion of the basis or evidence for the belief, the substitution of more realistic or helpful thoughts, and changing the relative's behaviour accordingly. For example, in the case of the relative who is fearful to leave the patient in the house alone (page 128), the catastrophic thinking behind this behaviour might include, 'If I leave him alone, something terrible could happen to him'. The therapist could help the relative to assess what is the basis or evidence for that belief. The relative's evidence might include, 'The doctor said he needs supervision; he made a suicide attempt three years ago; he's got no one else, so he needs me there.' Challenging or helping the relative to reconsider these factors could include discussing what aspects of his behaviour require supervision, and how much this necessitates the presence of the relative; what is his current suicide risk, and how the relative's presence reduces this risk; and what are the advantages and disadvantages for the patient and the relative of being always together. On the basis of the reviewed evidence, the relative might then be encouraged to test out the effects of leaving the patient alone, possibly for brief periods to begin with, and progressing in a graded manner for separations of increased duration, while assessing the benefits or disadvantages of the time spent apart from the patient. If the relative has given up many previously enjoyed activities, then work would also need to be done planning how the relative would spend time away from the home.

Changing Behavioural Responses

We have mentioned some of the critical and over-involved strategies, which are usually ineffective in resolving problems in the long term, as well as being associated with increased relapse risks for the patient, and often result in some considerable stress on the relative's part. Such responses are likely to be reported when problem-patient-focused situations are discussed, and alternative ways of responding to difficulties will need to be generated. Additionally, some relatives will not attempt, or will have stopped attempting, to actively cope or deal with problems, but will be very distressed by what the patient is or is not, doing or saying, and will seek guidance no how best to respond.

Helpful Behavioural Strategies for Responding to Behavioural Problems

Persistent Delusions and Hallucinations
Approximately one in four or five schizophrenia sufferers will experience persistent florid symptoms Chapter 9 gives practical guidelines for working with the patient to enhance their specific coping strategies. Where such a programme is available to the patient, the relative's co-operation may be not only a useful adjunct to the intervention, but also provide a means of educating the relative in appropriate coping responses, which will reduce their feelings of stress, triggered by the patient's delusional or hallucinatory talk and behaviour. For example, the relative can be informed of the coping responses the patient is encouraged to use, and may be able to prompt, reinforce, or otherwise assist the patient to use the techniques. In the earlier case example, increasing the husband's awareness of his wife's use of withdrawal helped him to respond more supportively, while reducing his own irritation (page 108).

Careful analysis of the patient's symptom behaviour and the family's response is necessary for planning how the relative might best support the patient's coping while reducing their own distress. All attempts to dissuade the patient of delusional ideas through arguments, threats, emotional appeals, and so on should be discouraged by helping the relative to see that these are ineffective in reducing symptoms – and may in fact increase the strength of delusional ideas – and are likely to increase the relative's own stress responses.

Similarly, colluding with the patient in the symptoms is an ineffective long-term strategy. Depending on the specific analysis of the problem, the relative may be encouraged to deliberately 'non-respond' to delusional talk (this is best rehearsed so that ignoring the behaviour is not felt to be a punitive response, for example, the mother of the son with persecutory delusions [page 108]); to distract the patient by starting a conversation about some everyday event; or to prompt the patient to engage in an alternative, distracting activity. Where such strategies do not decrease the symptom behaviour and the relative continues to feel distressed, he or she might be encouraged to withdraw from the patient, again in a non-punitive manner, or to reduce their exposure to situations where the patient is likely to evidence delusions or hallucinations.

Negative Symptoms
Chapter 7 gives guidelines for using a constructional approach to assist families to cope with deficit behaviours in patients. The behavioural responses appropriate for relatives will again depend on a careful analysis of the targeted problem, and the role relatives play in the carrying out of plans aimed to increase or promote positive functioning in the patient.

Aggression and Suicide Risk
Chapter 8 considers these two problems in more detail, and gives advice on the management of the problems in the family context.

Self-Management Techniques

Where there is a strong, affective component in the relative's response to the patient's behaviour, emotion-based coping strategies will probably be assessed to be an important emphasis for the intervention. Teaching the relative coping skills for managing their emotional responses – anxiety, depression, fear, irritation, and so on – will likely be necessary. Some of the cognitive strategies for assisting the relative to acquire more realistic and helpful interpretations of situations and behaviours have been discussed and illustrated in the case examples. In cases where the relative is assessed as having high levels of physiological anxiety, then applied relaxation training (Ost, 1987) may be appropriate. Where the relative has centred much of their life round the illness and has few pleasurable distractions, the use of goal-planning for meeting their own needs may be used (Chapter 7).

CONCLUSIONS

In this chapter we have provided guidelines for helping relatives to cope more effectively with difficult and stressful situations associated with the patient's illness. A detailed cognitive-behavioural analysis of specific situations, and a realistic appraisal of what combination of problem- and emotion-based coping strategies are appropriate, are important in determining the nature of individual interventions. It is often useful to address stress reduction in relatives before commencing interventions focused on directly increasing the patient's social functioning, but this is by no means inflexible; and, like the education component, stress management should be seen as an integral part of further work with the family.

Chapter 7

A Constructional Approach to Problems

As the primary focus of the stress management was to reduce stress and coping difficulties in relatives, so the chief aim of the goal-setting component is to assess and improve the social functioning of the patient. However, as there is considerable overlap between the two components, the therapist should not feel constrained to use only the goal setting when they have completed the stress management, or to apply stress management only to relatives' needs, and goal setting only for patients' needs. Moreover, some of the interventions to improve relatives' coping responses may result in improvements in the patient's functioning, and goal setting is often appropriate as an adjunct to stress management; improving the patient's functioning may also alleviate some of the stimuli or triggers of the relatives' stress responses. Additionally, stress management principles for relatives can be incorporated into many of the goal plans, and indeed may be an important aspect of the plan.

The approaches in this book have been compartmentalized largely for the sake of clarity, both in describing the range of intervention approaches and in emphasizing the dual goals of treatments: meeting the needs of relatives and the needs of patients. It is often most useful to target relative problems first by reducing stress and improving coping responses before assisting the relatives to help the patient more directly. This is due to a number of reasons. A high proportion of the relatives we worked with were acutely distressed at the commencement of the intervention, and it was felt more appropriate to reduce this distress by providing stress-management treatments before introducing them to rehabilitation strategies for the patient, which would make further demands on their resources. Also, many of the patients were recovering from an acute episode, and still had some positive symptoms and concentration difficulties in the early weeks; since the goal-setting sessions require some co-operation and participation from the patients, this would not have been possible.

We advise the therapist to tailor the interventions to the needs of the particular family they are working with, including a realistic appraisal of how easy or difficult it will be to improve the patient's functioning in the domestic setting by using approaches that are dependent on patient collaboration. The following general principles may be used in assessing the situation.

Where the patient is unable or unwilling to co-operate in discussing their needs, it is unadvisable to persist with goal-setting strategies aimed at affecting patient change through the collaboration of the whole family. 'Unable' or 'unwilling' might be operationalized as being unable to concentrate for at least 15 minutes in a discussion of current problems and issues. This situation may improve when, for example, the patient's clinical condition stabilizes through medication change, so it is important to continue to reassess the situation. It is not pointless to attempt psychological interventions with patients with drug-resistant, persistent symptoms, but methods need to be adapted to take account of the patient's inability to plan with the family (Chapter 9 gives details of work that can be done to help patients to cope with persistent symptoms; Chapter 6 suggests ways in which relatives might be involved in such work.) In some circumstances relatives can attempt goal setting to change patient behaviours without the active participation of the patient.

Where the relative(s) is/are continuing to have difficulties coping with day-to-day problems, it is more useful to target the main input to helping them to build better coping repertoires and attend to their own needs than to commencing rehabilitative work with the patient. Such relatives are characterized by high levels of anxiety and/or depression; often such relatives have few resources available to them, being socially isolated and restricted in their activites. The example of Mary in the preceding chapter (page 100) is such a situation. Most of the intervention input was targeted at her coping responses and at building her interests and social network, and goal-setting was used for her needs rather than for the patient's. Again, there should be flexibility in the approach, and some goal planning may be attempted later in the intervention with the patient.

More usually, three or four sessions are spent on relatives' stress management before commencing goal setting for patient needs. Stress management strategies are then monitored and reviewed at the beginning of each goal-setting session, and incorporated into the goal plans where necessary.

SOCIAL FUNCTIONING: ITS IMPORTANCE TO INTERVENTION PROGRAMMES

Aside from the worthwhile goal of improving the functioning of the patient, it has been suggested that promoting rehabilitative programmes within the family context is a powerful means of reducing the stress in the family environment. This makes a lot of sense: if one can directly improve the patient's situation by effectively restoring some of their functioning to a level closer to the premorbid level, then one reduces some of the problems and/or the stressors for the family members. In terms of the EE concepts, one effectively reduces or eliminates the opportunity for criticism or over-involved responses.

This line of thinking fits the available data from research: the successful intervention programmes have incorporated components with behavioural goal-setting approaches targeted at patient problems; it is difficult to assess how much of their success in reducing family tensions has come from this component *per se* (Kuipers *et al.*, 1988). There is also evidence that when patient behaviour improves, EE levels tend to fall, without recourse to intervention methods.

GOAL SETTING AND THE CONSTRUCTIONAL APPROACH

The goal setting and planning to be described aims to teach the family a constructional approach to the problems of family members. This entails construing problems as needs that might be best met through promoting positive behaviour change. It can be contrasted by what Schwartz and Goldiamond (1975) describe as the pathological approach, which focuses on the elimination of behaviours.

Essentially, in the face of presenting problems, the constructional approach asks the question, 'If the patient didn't have this problem, what would they be doing?', as opposed to the pathological question, 'How can we reduce or eliminate this behaviour?' This approach has two advantages in working with schizophrenic patients. Firstly, it focuses on the positive aspects of behaviour change in what sometimes seem to be an overwhelmingly negative set of circumstances; and secondly, by restating problems in positive terms, it allows the family members to begin to generate constructive solutions to problems. The key steps in the setting and planning of goals are listed in Table 7.1, and are described below; a case example later illustrates some of the main points.

ASSESSMENT

The chief assessment tool is a strengths/needs list, which is completed about the patient, but which may include the needs of other family members as well. The list tabulates on the one hand the patient's strengths, and on the other hand current difficulties/problems/issues/areas of

Table 7.1   Key Steps in Goal Setting and Planning

1. Identify difficulties/issues/problems/areas for change.
2. Translate problems into needs.
3. Identify strengths: abilities, interests, and resources.
4. Select a need on which to work.
5. Use the approaches to generate ways of meeting the need.
6. Set a realistic goal, and break this down into steps where appropriate.
7. Make a plan for each step (who does what, when, and how).
8. Review the goal or step.
9. Plan for maintenance, generalization, and extension of the goal.
10. Commence the new goal.

change. The latter are then translated into needs, using a constructional framework.

Strengths

These include the abilities, interests, and resources available to the patient. In later stages of the planning such strengths will be used to facilitate approaches to obtaining desired outcomes or treatment goals. Family members are encouraged to brainstorm strengths as a group, however, examples and prompts from the therapist's knowledge of the patient and his/her situation may often be required.

Frequently the patient's situation is dominated by a problem focus – the contrast between life before and after the illness – so that residual skills and abilities are not salient in the family members' thinking; or the family overlook abilities they perceive as too ordinary to mention, such as the ability to drive a car, or a particular work or leisure skill. Sometimes problems can be reconstrued in terms of strengths, for example, the other side of 'hardly ever goes out the house', is 'occasionally goes out to see a friend who lives nearby'; or, 'gets very irritable', can be translated as, 'has periods when controls temper'; and the problem, 'spends a lot of time alone in the bedroom' can be viewed as a positive coping strategy when used by the patient to reduce discomfort triggered by hallucinations.

When the patient is at a loss to suggest any interests, it may be useful to ask them to describe what they used to enjoy doing; a list of used-to-enjoy interests can then be added to the strengths.

Difficulties/Issues/Problems/Areas for Change

Family members, including the patient, are asked to complete this list. The patient is encouraged to include items pertaining to his relatives where these are important issues. This needs to be emphasized, for example, 'It is important that we get a good idea of the problems you are experiencing at home or elsewhere. These may include issues to do with your mother/father/wife/husband, etc., for example, things they do or say that are a problem to you, as well as the things that are mainly a problem to yourself.' Individual family members are encouraged to generate their own lists, and the lists are then pooled and information from earlier assessments, for example, from initial interviews or the FQ, are used by the therapist to identify further issues of concern.

Needs

Needs are a restatement of the problems in positive terms, using the constructional question, 'If the person didn't have this problem, what would he/she be doing?' One of the advantages of this process is that it immediately focuses the family's attention on what can be done about issues. For example, the problem 'Spends too much time lying around doing nothing', would be rephrased into something like, 'Needs to spend more time doing activities', or, 'Gets irritable' might be translated into 'Needs to learn to cope with irritability'.

Some examples of a strengths/needs list are given in Table 7.2.

At the end of the assessment session, relatives would be asked to take home their strengths/needs list and, if possible, add further items. The

Table 7.2 Example of a Strengths/Needs List and Goal Plan for a Teenage Girl Living With Her Parents

Strengths	Problems/Issues areas for change	Needs
Interests Music, clothes, reading, tennis, seeing friends, watching 'soaps' on TV. **Abilities** 'O' levels and good academic record at school, typing, driving license, cooking skills, good listener, enjoys helping others. **Resources** Parents, sister, and several friends and relatives keen to help; school helpful to assist her return.	*Parents won't leave me alone in house. *Worry about missing school. *Feeling tired and lethargic. *Overweight, spends a lot of time in bed, doing very little when up, avoiding friends and relatives, not interested in personal appreance.	1. Parents to discuss and plan to go out without daughter. 2. Return to school. 3. Review tiredness. 4. Reduce weight. 5. Get back to reasonable getting up/bedtimes. 6. Engage in more activities. 7. Get back to seeing friends/relatives. 8. Take more interest in personal appearance.

* Problems identified by the patient.

second session would then begin with the pooling of the relatives and patient's lists, before beginning targeting needs on which to work.

INTERVENTION STEPS

Selecting a Need on Which to Work

The needs of the family are reviewed and rank-ordered by the family in terms of priority and being realistic to achieve in the short term. It is important that the needs are seen as important to the patient, or are linked to other needs that have higher priority for him or her. For example, doing the housework may have priority for the relatives, whereas, in the case of a parental household, the patient may only be concerned with getting his or her own accommodation. The patient may see that say, improving, cooking skills would be an advantage and a step towards independent living, whereas cutting the grass may hold no interest or incentive.

Using the Approaches to Meet the Need

After identifying the need, the strengths list is scanned for approaches that might be used to meet it. At this stage the family are encouraged to brainstorm as much as possible. However tangential to the need strengths appear to be, there is a possibility they could be used. For each strength listed, the family can ask themselves, how might this be useful? For example, for a need of 'doing more activities', useful strengths could be interests the patient used to have, say, reading, music, sport.

Or, if the patient had difficulty getting started on things alone, they might think of people able to help if prosocial activities were required. The relevant strengths will help to shape the specific goal selected to work on.

Goal Setting

The needs that have been discussed are general and often non-specific, mapping out general areas for change, for example, 'do more activities'. Scanning the approaches will have helped to decide on a more precise change target; for example, activities arising out of the patient's interests, abilities, and resources would have been generated from the strengths in examining the need 'to do more activities'.

A goal or outcome can next be set, which is stated in clear behavioural terms: such a goal must allow for attainment to be assessed; in other words, it must be expressed in terms of observable behaviour. In selecting goals, it is best to start with ones that stand a good chance of being achieved in a relatively short time period, that is, one or two weeks. This will provide the family with immediate feedback and reinforcement of their efforts.

Goals that set new behaviours at a level not far from the patient's existing repertoire are more likely to be achieved, as are ones that build on the strengths. For example, if a patient currently does not get up until midday, it would be better to aim for him/her to rise by say, 10:30a.m. and to build in a range of preferred activities the patient can do when they get up as incentives. Expecting the patient to start getting up at 8:30a.m. to go to a day-centre they dislike attending is a goal doomed to failure, however specific the objective.

Where necessary, the goal can be broken down into steps that can be achieved in a week or so, and which are relatively simple to accomplish. Again, each step should be specified in terms of observable behaviour. Not all the steps need to be planned at the outset; a first step can be planned and progress reviewed before deciding on the next step.

The Plan

It is important that the plan for each step specifies who does what, when and how, with whom, and with how much help. The relatives' and patient's participation in each goal step should be specified and, if necessary, rehearsed. It will often be necessary to incorporate prompts into the execution of plans, and to maximize the reinforcing value of achieving goal steps: a common difficulty for patients is in initiating behaviour, and the patient may feel the effort required to perform a task may not be equal to the subjective value of the goal.

Where used, prompts need to be discussed and rehearsed. It is sometimes best for the patient to take responsibility for the prompts by, for example, using written reminders to do tasks or to go places, which can be posted in prominent places. Similarly, rehearsal of the advantages versus the disadvantages of performing tasks with the patient may be a useful method of initiating behaviours, and these advantages can be written down for the patient to review at home. We have successfully used this method in planning ways of helping the patient to get out of bed, to perform tasks, or to get places on time.

Where family members are used as prompters, it is important that this is acceptable to the patient and that the relative is able to perform the prompting in an acceptable way, that is, in a neutral and age-appropriate manner; a prompt can easily sound like a nag, or at least be construed as one. Details of the plan need to be agreed by all the participants. The role of the relatives should be carefully considered, particularly where relatives have demonstrated intrusive, over-protective, or critical re-

sponses in similar circumstances in the past. Sometimes the direct pro-
gramming of a passive role for relatives may be necessary: just to stand
back and allow the patient to carry out the plan, or, where further help is
needed, to try and find a friend or less-involved relative to carry out the
prompts and assistance.

Where the family is isolated, it may be necessary for the therapist to
carry out roles in order to help the patient to initiate behaviours. For
example, in one case, the first step in the patient's goal to work as a
volunteer in a centre for elderly people was to visit the centre and to meet
the staff. The patient failed to turn up for his appointment, reporting that
he had got ready to go, but felt too nervous and had stayed at home.
Reviewing the step, his mother offered to go with him the next time the
meeting was arranged, but the patient felt it was inappropriate for a man
in his mid-20s to be accompanied by his mother, and this was supported
by the therapist. In the absence of other social supporters, the therapist
arranged to meet the patient at the centre, and to stay with him for a
short period. This minimal support was sufficient for the patient to carry
out the step and continue with the plan. In such cases, unless the
therapist is able to make a long-term commitment, it is important they
quickly fade out of the plan, otherwise they will be artificially supporting
the patient's behaviour in a way that cannot be maintained in the long
term.

Writing out the plan with a copy for each participant is worthwhile,
including details of dates and times where tasks are to be carried out.
Some steps may require repeated practice before the patient feels able to
move on to the next step. Issues to be considered are balancing the need
for the patient to perceive real progress against pushing forward too
quickly and risking failure. It is well worth spending time to cover all
eventualities, including some advance trouble-shooting, or what happens
if the planned outcome is not achieved. For example, if the wife prompts
her husband, the patient, that they have agreed to go out for a meal that
evening, and he declines saying he is not up to it since he feels too agitated,
what then? It is better that such issues are discussed before the events. A
strategy for the husband to cope with his agitation may be written into
the plan, and the wife may be able to offer her husband reassurance that
they have selected a quiet restaurant and have agreed only to go out for
one hour.

It may be necessary to review coping responses necessary for the
relative. For example, if the plan involves the patient doing a task independently and the relative is concerned that this will put the patient at
risk, then the risks need to be discussed and strategies for dealing with
worries rehearsed. In the earlier stages of goal planning it is best if the
family do not persist with a step that they repeatedly fail to achieve

despite following the planned procedure, but discuss the problems at the next session with the therapist. An atmosphere of experimentation should be developed through statements such as, 'We seem to have covered most eventualties in planning this step for our goal. Try to follow all the planning we have made, but don't worry if things don't turn out. This only means that we hadn't considered all aspects of the plan – sometimes things are different when you try them out – and that we need to get together and think again.'

Reviewing the Goal

At the next session, progress with the goal step is reviewed; efforts reinforced; goals changed, abandoned, or new steps commenced. If the goal or step was written in clear behavioural terms, then it is easy for everyone to assess the outcome. In cases where the step or goal was not achieved, then an analysis of what went wrong with the plan should be made. Partial successes should be emphasized and reinforced. Any failure to achieve the goals should be viewed as a planning failure, since one otherwise risks reducing the low self-efficacy of the patient and further diminishing their motivation, and also possibly making the relatives feel the patient 'is not trying'.

It is important to keep some form of progress record, with either the therapist, or preferably the patient or family member, taking responsibility for recording progress. This might take the form of a simple diary of goals, with dates of achieving steps, partially achieving steps, or abandoning goals. Obtaining from the patient estimates of the ease/difficulty of performing each goal step – for example, using a scale of 0 (very easy) to 10 (very difficult) – can be useful: even small increases in ease of accomplishing tasks can be fed back to the patient to emphasize progress when they feel they are not making much headway. The ratings also can be helpful in assisting the therapist and family to understand the subjective difficulty of tasks, and whether plans need to be modified to make goals easier to accomplish.

Maintenance, Generalization, and Extensions of the Goal

Once the patient has achieved a targeted goal, it is important to plan for maintenance, and/or to attempt to generalize the success to other specified activities and situations. Take for example the goal of attending an evening class at an adult education college. Once the goal has been achieved – say the patient has gone to the class for two or three consecutive weeks – and the ratings indicate the patient finds it fairly easy to attend, it is useful to troubleshoot any reasons the patient might have in sustaining attendance. What is the patient getting out of attending? What difficulties does he/she experience? How might any problems be overcome?

For generalization, situations similar to the targeted goal might be suggested by the patient and/or family members. For example, if the patient has succeeded in visiting a friend where previously they avoided leaving the house, what other places of similar ease or difficulty might they go to? Interests from the strengths list might be incorporated into the planning of outings, and the goal might be extended by planning for outings involving longer distances from home, or incorporating other needs of the patient.

EXAMPLE OF A GOAL PLAN

Background

Peter has had schizophrenic symptoms since age 16. He was 18 at the time of the intervention, and had recently been discharged after his third hospital admission. At that time he was not reporting auditory hallucinations, which were present during the hospital admission, but continued to have persecutory delusions concerning the devil. He had a school history of low academic achievement, and had had no employment since leaving school. He lived with his mother, Irene. He spent most of the day in bed, feeling too 'frightened' to leave the flat alone. His mother was anxious about leaving him in the flat alone since he had made an attempt to cut his wrists six months previously, and she had reduced her own social activities accordingly. He had frequent outbursts of temper directed at his mother. They lived in a two-bedroom council flat on a high-rise estate, and finances were tight. Peter's mother was divorced and Peter had very little contact with his father although he lived in the same town. Irene was in regular contact with her sister and her elder married son, and had a relationship with a man, John, who she saw several times a week.

Stress Management

Irene had been taking tranquilizers prescribed by her GP since the onset of Peter's illness. Early interviewing had revealed that Irene had a very confused idea of the nature of Peter's illness, had problems

Goal Setting

Assessment

A strengths/needs list for Peter was established.

Strengths	Problems/Issues/Change areas	Needs
Able to stay alone in flat for short periods.	Lacks friends and social contacts. Difficulty mixing with people.	To mix with people.
Able to and enjoys looking round local market alone.	Spends long periods doing nothing.	To increase activities.
	Rarely leaves the flat. Unable to travel alone on buses.	To get out more.
Positive symptoms much improved.	Not attending day-care.	
Temper outbursts less frequent.	Temper outbursts.	To learn to control temper.
Willing and able to do some housework and jobs in the flat.	Easily irritated.	
People who are willing to help: brother, aunt, John, a friend Mark who lives locally, mother.	Bored a lot of the time.	To occupy time with interests.
	Poor concentration.	To improve concentration.

Used to enjoy talking to people.
Good at drawing.
Enjoys reading.
Enjoys listening to music.
Likes TV.
Likes to look good and dress well.
Used to play football.
Used to do weight training.

Has a place at a day-centre and would like to attend.
Has a bus pass.

coping with his symptoms, and was significantly anxious and mildly depressed. The stress management sessions had highlighted Peter's temper outbursts as her main current concern (the interventions used are described in Chapter 8). The interventions were successful in reducing the frequency and severity of the temper outbursts, and Irene established a daily break of time away from Peter.

Selecting a Need to Work on

Both Irene and Peter felt that a need of high priority was for Peter to get out of the flat more often. It was felt this overlapped with several of his other needs, for example, to increase his activities, and that in order to see more people and to attend day-care he would have to be able to travel independently. Also it would be helpful for Irene if she had more time to herself.

Using Approaches to Meet the Need

A number of strengths were relevant to the need. There was evidence that Peter could already go short distances from the house unaccompanied, and was able to go on a bus if someone went with him. The relatives and friends he knew in the town would be useful people to go and visit, and/or might be able to help with a plan, e.g., by accompanying him on some journeys.

Setting a Goal

The mother and patient were guided to set a goal that might be accomplished in a few weeks. It was decided that the goal should involve getting a bus to visit someone, and Peter selected his brother, since he was already in regular contact with him and felt comfortable talking to him. Also, he lived on a nearby bus route. Peter was keen to try to achieve the goal as soon as possible, but a careful analysis of the possible difficulties for him indicated he would need some help in the early stages, and that it would be better to attempt the goal by working through a series of graded steps. Since Peter was already able to travel with someone accompanying him, it was suggested that he should start at this level, with help travelling to and from his brother's house, and that this might then be withdrawn if all went well. The final goal would be to travel to Mathew's house and back by bus twice a week, unaccompanied. Goal steps suggested were: 1. To travel to Mathew's house and back by bus, accompanied. 2. To travel . . . accompanied on the bus journey there, but return by bus alone. 3. To travel . . . by bus there and back unaccompanied.

The Plan (Who Should Do What, When, and Where)

When the journey should take place. A factor to consider was when Peter felt best able to make the journey. He ruled out going in the evening, since he felt concerned about who might be on the estate at night, which was a realistic problem since fights and muggings were commonplace. He felt afternoon was his best time, as he felt more tired and tense in the mornings. Since his brother worked, this meant the visits would have to take place at weekends.

Who would accompany him. It was felt that it would be difficult for anyone but his mother to make the time commitment to accompanying Peter. Strategies for encouraging him on the journey were rehearsed. Peter's concerns focused around people thinking he looked 'strange', and coping self-statements were suggested such as, 'Everyone looks at other people. If people look at me this is unlikely to be because I look strange,' 'In order to stop thinking about other people, I can concentrate on what everything looks like on the bus route. I can look at the colour of the houses, how many people I see, what make of cars there are on the road, and so on.' It was agreed that his mother would prompt him to use these statements and strategies on the journey.

The content of the visit. Peter was concerned that he had nothing to say to anyone. Some brainstorming was done as to how interactions could be made easier. Ideas included sharing an activity such as a job in the house, or listening to music, or doing some local shopping. He was encouraged to discuss these ideas with Mathew before his visit.

It was decided a preliminary step should be introduced into the plan to phone Mathew, tell him about the goal, arrange the first visit, and to discuss what they might do during the visit.

Review of the Plan

The next session reviewed how Peter had got on with steps 1 and 2. The first step had been successful, and the visit had been arranged for the Saturday when the plan was for Peter to go with Mathew to buy a record, and then help with some gardening. The second step was also achieved, and Peter had felt pleased with the visit. However, there had been some trouble between Peter and his mother on the way there, and Peter had argued with her and said he did not want her to walk with

him. Irene had been distressed by this, not knowing whether to leave
Peter to make the journey alone, or whether she should stay in case he
felt unable to make the bus journey. She had in fact stayed with him.
There had been no problems on the return journey, and John, Irene's
friend, had offered to accompany Peter on subsequent trips. Both Peter
and Irene felt this was a better alternative, and it was decided that Peter
would repeat the second step with John accompanying him the following
week. This was successful, and at Peter's suggestion partial accompani-
ment was omitted, and Peter completed his goal of travelling to and from
the visit unaccompanied within three weeks of commencing the goal
steps.

Maintenance and Generalization of the Goal

Although the goal of visiting Mathew was successfully achieved, Peter
felt he wanted to see other people besides his brother, and that weekly
visits to Mathew were probably too frequent in the long term. Without
the use of goal setting, he had started to go to the local shop several times
a week, and time was spent helping him to set other goals for visits to his
friend's and to John's house. These were not broken down into steps; he
was able to use buses without difficulty, and the main function of the
goals was to help him programme his day and evaluate his progress.

Further detailed plans were used for day-care attendance, but despite initial success in achieving the goal of independent travelling and
attendance, this was not maintained. Peter felt he did not get on with
people at the centre, that they were mainly a lot older than him, and the
activities were not of interest to him. Later stages of the intervention
involved organizing alternative daytime activities at a drop-in centre for
teenagers, and Peter later moved into supported hostel accomodation.

SOME ISSUES AND PROBLEMS IN THE USE OF GOAL PLANNING

We noted earlier the importance of understanding why patients and
relatives are unable to carry out agreed plans. One problem can be that
the perceived benefits to the patient do not match the effort necessary
to achieve the goal. Low rewards can be increased by, for example,
including some self-reward contingent on completing a task, or by rehearsing with the patient the benefits in achieving a goal or step and
writing advantages down so the patient can refer to them at home: be it
these might be improved mood, self-confidence, access to other more
rewarding activities, and so on. We have successfully used the latter

strategies in plans that required a lot of effort from patients where the immediate pay-off was low; for example, getting out of bed earlier.

Sometimes the reason for non-completion of goals is that the task set was too difficult: the gap between the patient's present and new behaviour was too large. One problem is in achieving a reasonable balance between setting goals that are meaningful to the patient, yet are not too difficult to achieve. 'Difficult' may mean demanding too much physical activity, concentration, social contact, planning, decision-making, or other skills. Each task and its associated requirements need to be analyzed when problems occur, and it may be necessary to help the patient to acquire some anxiety management, social or other coping skills in order to help them to attain desired goals.

Sometimes goals and plans are agreed during sessions, but are not carried out because family members have doubts about their usefulness or validity. For example, Donald lived with his parents, who were both in their 70s. His mother's concern was that Donald lay on the lounge settee for hours on end, making no contribution to household tasks, which was particularly problematic since his father was disabled and unable to do housework either. An agreed goal was for Donald to clean his own room each week, which involved some prompting from his mother. However, the family reported they had not carried out the plan. Although Donald had offered to clean his room, his mother had said it was not important, and 'it wasn't really man's work'. Further discussion focused on what tasks were more appropriate for Donald to carry out; mainly those that would meet his need of increasing his activities while sharing some of the domestic work. It was agreed he should decorate the kitchen, and over a period of several weeks he successfully achieved this goal.

Obtaining some consensus among family members as to what constitutes a problem in the household is not always straightfoward. As in the example above, failure to contribute to the housework, or untidiness, are often issues in households where the patient is lethargic and spends a lot of time lying around the house. One family member may be pre-occupied with thinking about the untidiness of the patient, whereas the patient themself and other relatives may think this to be fairly unimportant.

One way of at least facilitating some useful discussion of the matter is to encourage relatives and the patient to translate the problem into positive and specific behaviours, for example, what the patient would be doing if he/she were more tidy, be it clean their room, wash their clothes, or whatever, and then generate the pros and cons of working towards a positive change. The pros might include helping the concerned relative to feel less irritated and thus improve their relationship with the patient; there would be less work for whoever has to clean the mess of the patient, with some spin-off for the patient at least in terms of reduced arguments in the household, if not in terms of more positive personal benefit. The most likely negative consequence would be the effort required to tidy up, wash, or whatever the specific tasks involve. Another helpful strategy is to try and find a household task for the patient to complete that is acceptable to the patient and the concerned family member.

It is important not to lose sight of the fact that some problems associated with the illness, particularly when it has a severe and chronic course, may continue indefinitely, for example, persistent and drug-resistent symptoms, the inability of the patient to resume their former occupational level, or to establish or maintain many friendships and social activities, or to live without considerable support. Although for most patients some positive change will be possible, and realistic goals can be confidently selected to work on, when the problem itself cannot be significantly reduced, some of the issues raised by relatives will require emotion-based coping (Chapter 6).

Goal Setting to Meet Relatives' Needs

Although the examples in this chapter have focused on the use of goal setting and planning procedures in the context of meeting the rehabilitative needs of patients, the format is equally useful in tackling the needs of relatives, particularly when they have reduced their occupational and recreational interests and social contacts as a consequence of the illness.

A desired aim of goal setting with family members is that they will achieve independence in using the format to plan for positive change. Initially, the therapist works through the processes with the family, and later encourages them to select needs, focus on strengths, set specific goals, and work out plans to achieve the objectives. However, there is considerable variation in how autonomous families become in planning positive-rehabilitative strategies, and a considerable number may need prolonged, if not indefinite, support from the therapist. It would be misleading to create an impression that if all the guidelines in this text are followed, then success is guaranteed and all patients will make significant progress. On the other hand, the approach has sufficient flexibility to be adaptable to the situations of most schizophrenic patients living with relatives. Its chief advantages lie in the focus on positive change rather than problem reduction; the utilization of existing strengths; the attempts to minimize failure through planning for intermediate goals; and the easy evaluation of outcomes. In the majority of families we worked with, particularly when the illness was episodic and the patient was not suffering from continuous positive symptoms, most of the key problems were worked through over a period of four to six months, and often the patient thereafter was able to continue planning their won goals with limited help and encouragement from the therapist, family, friends, or other resource agents.

Chapter 8

Issues of Engaging and Maintaining Family Involvement

Previous chapters have outlined the principles of interventions with families, and have attempted to give specific advice on how some of the needs of relatives and patients may be addressed through educational, stress management, and constructional goal-setting approaches. We have drawn the reader's attention to some of the common difficulties in carrying out interventions, and to suggested ways of analyzing and working through potential problems. However, as there is enormous variation in the severity and chronicity of the problems families present, we have selected the engagement and maintainence of the family in treatment as an area of difficulty for further consideration.

ENGAGEMENT AND MAINTENANCE OF THE FAMILY IN TREATMENT

Despite the encouraging results to support the benefits of family intervention programmes, clinicians attempting to implement such a programme may be surprised to find that families do not always receive the intervention with similar enthusiasm. Intervention studies have reported that a number of families either refused to participate in the intervention or withdrew from treatment. The range of families refusing intervention is 7–35%; the range of families withdrawing from treatment is 7–50%; and there is a total non-compliance range of 8–50%. A follow-up study of 'inclusion refusers', 'treatment refusers', and 'drop-outs' from the Salford Study indicated that 12 out of 18 (67%) of these patients relapsed in the subsequent nine months. These results suggest not only that some patients and their families are difficult to engage and maintain in treatment, but that this group may be at elevated risk of recurrent relapse (Smith *et al.*, 1990; Tarrier, 1991b). There is also evidence that such a patient population makes a heavy financial demand on the mental health services (Hafner *et al.*, 1989). If research results are to be translated into clinical practice in an effective and economical manner, the engagement and maintenance of families in treatment is a crucial factor.

Explanatory models of adherence and health behaviour have emphasized a cost-benefit, decision-making perspective – that is, the patient makes a decision whether to initiate or stay in treatment based upon a balance of the perceived costs and benefits. This analysis can be translated to the engagement and adherence of families in family interventions. The family's participation will be dependent on the perceived susceptability to the illness (in this case, the likelihood of the patient suffering a relapse); the perceived effectiveness of the preventative measures (the estimated efficacy of the intervention in reducing the patient's relapse risk); and the perceived costs (physical, psychological, and economical to the patient and/or the family). This analysis focuses on the relatives' cognitive processes in coming to a decision concerning participation. The implications for the engagement and maintenance of the family in treatment are, firstly, that these cognitive processes need to be acknowledged and assessed; and, secondly, adherence can be facilitated by taking action that will maximize the predicted benefits of the intervention and decrease the costs. For example, consider the following case:

Mrs Brown was a woman in her late 30s who had been hospitalized for her third acute episode of schizophrenia. After three weeks in hospital, she was free from schizophrenic symptoms, having responded well to medication. It was planned to discharge her back to her family home, where she lived with her husband and two children, aged 14 and 12.

When first approached, Mr Brown accepted the request to discuss his wife's illness with the psychologist, and was co-operative in completing the RAI. Ha also attended two information sessions which attempted to modify some of his beliefs about his wife's problems. Mr Brown had been upset by the fact that his wife had made a serious suicide attempt prior to her hospital admission. At this stage, he was worried about the reasons for his wife's suicidal behaviour, and was concerned that she might not fully recover. He was unaware of the delusional thinking behind much of her disturbed behaviour at home, and had felt that her neglect of the housework and childcare was a cause rather than a consequence of the illness. His principal strategies when difficulties arose were to get at her to do more housework, and when she became acutely ill, he avoided being with her as much as possible.

When Mrs Brown was discharged home, her husband's attitude to further involvement with the psychologist changed. He was reluctant to plan for further appointments, saying that he did not see the point since his wife was now well. Attempts to persuade Mr Brown to maintain some involvement with the therapist met with resistance. Why should he participate, since he was not the one who was sick? Furthermore, if she did become ill again, then it was Mr Brown's view that 'the hospital should take care of her. If she still needs treatment now, then she should stay in hospital till she is better and doesn't need treatment.'

An attempt was made to leave the family's options open by arranging to visit the family at home to review Mrs Brown's progress. During the first visit Mr Brown was reasonably co-operative in discussing his wife's progress in general terms, but soon disengaged himself by sitting with his back to the therapists and watching television.

Problems with the engagement of Mr Brown in an intervention programme seemed to include his beliefs about the illnesses. Despite the educational input Mr Brown had received, he did not accept the importance of his own role, or other environmental factors, in supporting his wife's well-being; nor did he make a connection with the stresses at home and his wife's relapses. Moreover, he felt that when his wife recovered from her acute illnesses, then his worries were over, thus there was no need for him to seek out further advice or information. Essentially, he felt that schizophrenia, like physical illness, was mainly treated by doctors in hospitals. To increase his co-operation, it would be necessary to demonstrate to him that he and his family could significantly benefit from the psychologist's input, with little cost or effort from himself.

FACTORS AFFECTING ENGAGEMENT AND MAINTENANCE IN TREATMENT

Meichenbaum and Turk (1987) have summarized the factors affecting adherence to treatment into five general categories: characteristics of the client; characteristics of the treatment regimen; features of the disease; the relationship between the health-care provider and the client; and the clinical setting. There is considerable overlap between these categories, but the headings provide a useful framework in which to discuss some of the sources of difficulty in engaging and maintaining the families of schizophrenic patients in treatment.

Characteristics of the Client

In discussing the client in this instance we are referring to the patient's relatives and family, and not the index patient.

Physical Health and Age of the Relative

Many families consist of elderly parents and their schizophrenic son or daughter. With age, the relative has an increased risk of poor physical health, and participation in an intervention programme over a long period of time may be difficult in the absence of special considerations. Such special considerations may include the timing and location of appointments, as well as the provision of written instructions to help with the retention of advice. Additionally, some older clients may have become socially isolated, and have few social supports or means of spending time away from close contact with the son or daughter, and will require help in addressing these difficulties.

Competing Demands and Lack of Resources

There may be other competing demands, such as employment commitments, caring for young children, problematic social and emotional relationships; or the lack of resources, such as money, transport, or time, which makes adherence difficult, especially if sessions take place in the hospital during normal working hours.

Comment

The costs to the family of participation in an intervention programme can be decreased if a range of options in terms of localities and timing of sessions are made available. For example, the choice of the sessions taking place in the family home, local health centre, perhaps with child-care facilities or the hospital, with a flexibility of hours to accommodate relatives with work commitments. It is unrealistic to insist that all relatives attend all sessions if work or other commitments make this problematic. Possibly one key relative can attend regularly, with others attending less frequently, and the 'primary' relative can be helped to communicate the content of sessions to other members.

Lack of Understanding About the Illness or Inappropriate or Conflicting Health Beliefs

These may be idiosyncratic, sociocultural, or ethnic conceptualizations of the disease and its treatment. In Chapter 5 we discussed how the relatives' perceptions of the patient's problems and their cause may conflict with the professionals' explanatory model, and we emphasized the importance of understanding how relatives' beliefs can mediate their coping responses. The chapters on stress management and goal setting (Chapters 6 and 7) illustrate how cognitions can present blocks for changing management strategies, and ways of helping relatives to reappraise and reattribute behaviours. Conflicting explanations held by the relatives can be dealt with in a manner similar to incorrect causal explanations held by sufferers of emotional disorders (Hawton *et al.*, 1989). The differing explanations held by the professional and relative are acknowledged, and evidence is gathered to support or refute the alternatives. The influence of cultural factors, especially relating to minority and ethnic groups, are probably an important, but as yet unknown, variable.

Apathy and Pessimism

Particularly where the illness is longstanding, with unremitting symptoms and the patient functioning at a low level, despite the best efforts of the family there may be a feeling of hopelessness. With such problems the family may be reluctant to co-operate at the outset, or difficulties may arise when agreed strategies are not carried out because relatives do not feel their efforts will result in any meaningful change. Sometimes it is possible to gain the co-operation of relatives by placing the emphasis on their own needs through stress management programmes, or the increased use of services by the patient, for example, day-care attendance. However, working towards the patient moving out of home may be a more appropriate option in some cases, with rehabilitative goals in the home directed to this final outcome.

Residential Instability

Sometimes the patient is unpredictable in his or her residence with the family. In such cases it may be possible to work with the relatives alone.

Comment

Intervention programmes should be flexible, and be able to respond to the identified and prioritized needs of either the relative or the patient as required. This may mean addressing the mood of the relative or the functioning of the patient by medication changes; or psychological help with symptom management; or looking for alternatives, such as day-care or alternative housing, that will help reduce family burden. Demonstrating the possibility of change in the short term may be necessary to increase the relatives' belief in long-term change; in the early stages, using interventions that are less dependent on family co-operation may provide a foot in the door to later working directly with the relatives.

Characteristics of the Individual

Dispositional characteristics of the relative, frequently summarized as poor motivation, are often cited to explain lack of adherence to intervention programmes, even though such explanations frequently lack conceptual clarity and empirical support. The relatives' level of EE has also been used to explain their low level of co-operation with the mental health services. However, it is possible that the relationship between EE and low levels of co-operation are the result of some third factor, such as aversive experiences with the mental health services. An analysis of the factors contributing to poor compliance is likely to be a more fruitful method of generating possible solutions, rather than attributing a lack of success to characteristics in the family members – although blaming the family is an easier option for therapists.

A further difficulty in working with families is the assumption of a simple deficit model: relatives have knowledge and skills deficits, and the intervention aims to give them the information they do not have, and to teach them new coping skills. This assumption can potentially alienate relatives, who rightly may feel they have the practical experience of coping with schizophrenia, since they have been living with the patient for a long time. To engage such relatives it is necessary to acknowledge their expertise, and to put forword professional advice as a complementary type of knowledge, the combination of which will form the basis of the collaborative endeavour.

Dissatisfaction With the Practitioner or Treatment

There is no direct evidence that relatives fail to enter family interventions because they are dissatisfied with the therapist or the approach, however, this may be a factor affecting early drop-out. Similarly, negative experiences with other aspects of the mental health services may act as a negative 'halo' effect. Nelson *et al.* (1975) found that the single most influential variable in schizophrenic patients' drug default was the patient's assessment of his physician's interest in him; a perception of interest and a clear and adequate explanation of the intervention are important variables in engaging relatives.

One of the advantages of using a lengthy semistructured interview procedure such as the CFI or RAI is that it allows the relative considerable time to talk and to feel they are being listened to; it is sometimes the first occasion any professional has listened to their views and concerns for such an extended time period. The more common experience of interviews with mental health professionals is a matter of obtaining information, with little feedback or exploration of personal concerns. The lengthy assessment procedures we describe provide an opportunity to build rapport, which can be further strengthened if the therapist is accessible to the family. Good rapport with the family may be partly due to a contrast effect with past negative experiences.

Relatives' Expectations and Attitudes Towards Treatment

Relatives who expect and want something completely at odds to the treatment offered will be difficult to engage and maintain. One potential recruit to the Salford project wanted her daughter confined to an institution as she had been told previously by another psychiatrist this was an option. She refused to consider any alternative, and terminated all further contact will all services once she realized this was no longer a realistic possibility. Here there is a clear conflict between the needs of the patient and the needs of the relative, or at least those as defined by herself. In this case, attitudes to treatment may be related to attitudes towards the patient.

Liaison with other professional and non-professional agencies to inform and update them about the nature and goals of family intervention may help to avoid misunderstandings about the programme. It is certainly worth investing time in talking to consumer and support groups.

CHARACTERISTICS OF TREATMENT

In adhering to an intervention programme, the subject is required to initiate and maintain a new set of behaviours. It would seem probable that the greater the contrast between the relative's established behaviour and the new behaviour, and the longer the former has been established, the greater difficulty the relative will have in adhering to the intervention programme. The literature also suggests that the more complex and intrusive the treatment regimen the lower the adherence. Furthermore, adherence generally deteriorates over time; continued adherence over time is especially important in family management of a chronic disorder such as schizophrenia, in which the patient is sensitive to environmental stress.

These characteristics of the intervention – contrast, complexity, and intrusiveness – may affect the relatives' adherence, especially over extended periods of time. Intervention strategies should aim to gradually shape the relatives' behaviour to an increasingly closer approximation of the desired behaviour, and organize the contingencies to maintain these newly acquired behaviours. In the case example of Mr Brown (page 137), the husband who did not wish to participate in intervention sessions, by scheduling intervention sessions at home while he was present, it was possible to obtain his co-operation in at least reviewing his wife's progress, at little cost to himself. Over a number of sessions he increased his participation in the discussions about selecting the goals his wife might work towards. From merely commenting on his wife's behaviour he began to offer advice or opinions about how she might increase her social activities outside the home; cope more effectively with the children; and, later, obtain part-time employment. However, over a nine month period it was never possible to obtain his full participation, nor to get him to contract to any systematic changes in his own behaviour, and there remained difficulties in communication between the couple, and regular disagreements that focused on Mrs Brown's neglect of the housework.

Disease or Disorder Variables

Acute Crisis

Studies that have attempted to recruit families during remission or periods of stable community tenure have reported great difficulties in engagement (Cheek *et al.*, 1971; Hudson, 1975). Families appear more amenable to help during critical periods such as hospital admission or symptom relapse. Similarly, rapid remission of symptoms following discharge can be associated with decreased adherence or termination of the intervention, since the family no longer perceives the necessity for further intervention. In such cases, where the families drop out of active intervention, contact with the family can be maintained through progress monitoring sessions, so that access back into the intervention is available if required.

Chronic Course

The families of patients experiencing a chronic illness with severe deficits may feel their actions have no influence on the patient, and hence view the situation as impossible to change.

Disruptive, Aggressive, and Violent Behaviour

Aggressive and violent behaviour is one of the problems relatives find most difficult to cope with. Relatives of very disturbed or violent patients may not be prepared to participate in an intervention programme for a number of reasons: if the patient is relatively stable the relatives may fear upsetting the status quo, or they may be too frightened of the patient participating. The latter occurred in the Salford project when a young woman who wanted to participate declined intervention because she was too frightened of the reactions of her violent father.

Comment

Although intervention should always be on offer, even to patients with a chronic illness, the chances of successful adherence and management are probably increased the earlier the intervention is implemented in the patient's illness. Furthermore, the critical periods when engagement and drop-out are more probable should be recognized and planned for.

Family interventions cannot exist in isolation, and should be part of a comprehensive and integrated mental health service, which has a range of options that can potentially meet families with special needs. For example, the confidence of relatives in dealing with violent patients will probably be increased if they can call on services which will reliably respond with advice, emotional support, or practical help.

In general, moderate levels of aggressive and disruptive behaviour can be successfully reduced by the clear setting of limits of what is permissible and what is not, and the consistent application of management strategies within this context (pages 146–153).

The Relationship Between the Family and the Mental Health Service

Dissatisfaction and Stigmatization

Numerous surveys have shown that families express dissatisfaction with their interaction with mental health personnel (Bernheim, 1989; Lefley, 1989), complaining they are unable to obtain information from professionals who have a major role in caring for the patient. Families also report frustrations in attempting to obtain answers to reasonable questions, and in receiving reluctant and sometimes hostile communications from mental health workers. There is evidence that the benefits of educating relatives are not in the acquisition of knowledge itself, but in the non-specific effects of reducing anxiety, worry, and perceived burden. The lack of access to information, therefore, is likely to exacerbate these emotional problems.

Theories of family pathogenesis have in the past been widespread and are still held by some professionals (Bernheim, 1989). This has resulted in relatives being blamed and stigmatized for the patient's illness. More recently, the term 'High Expressed Emotion' has been used erroneously and spuriously to label relatives who are distressed, concerned, or 'difficult' (McIntyre *et al.*, 1989). Being blamed for causing the illness, or being treated with neglect has resulted, not unreasonably, in relatives becoming dissatisfied with mental health professionals, and sometimes avoiding contact with them.

The willingness of families to engage in new intervention programmes will be determined by their previous experience with other mental health professionals. Unpleasant or negative experiences, especially during the potentially emotional circumstances of hospital admission, may result in the general rejection of all mental health services – the negative 'halo' effect. Negative attitudes and behaviours of staff towards relatives may result in relatives becoming increasingly anxious and worried about the patient or overly protective towards them, which could lead to a decrease in the relatives' effective coping.

Differing Priorities

Several studies have indicated that patients and their relatives have different priorities to those of staff (MacCarthy *et al.*, 1986; McIntyre *et al.*, 1989). Clearly, if problems and their solutions are viewed with differing levels of importance by families and therapists then adherence will be jeopardized, and it is therefore important to elicit what patients and relatives view as their high-priority needs before embarking on intervention goals. This is one of the rationales for the family to generate a problem/areas-of-change list at the beginning of the stress management (Chapter 6) and goal-setting exercises (Chapter 7). It is sometimes the case, however, that there are problems with patients and relatives seeing selected goals as unimportant to their real areas of concern, even when such goals have been the subject of collaborative discussion, which is sometimes the reason for plans being abandoned by the family members.

Clinic and Service Variables

The organization of the mental health clinic or service may have a strong influence on adherence. Characteristics such as the nature and location of the treatment setting; a long waiting time; individual appointments; duration of appointments; clinic opening times; difficulty accessing the service when required; lack of cohesiveness of the treatment service; continuity of personnel; responsiveness of the clinical service, may all directly or indirectly affect adherence.

In general, if clinical services were organized with more attention to consumer's needs, there would probably be an increase both in consumer satisfaction and adherence. In particular, the use of appropriate verbal reminders, prompts, telephone calls and follow-up letters to target appointment attendance and the completion of homework exercises could be incorporated into the intervention programme to good effect.

Chapter 9

The Problems of Violence and Suicide Risk

AGGRESSION AND VIOLENCE

One of the most difficult problems relatives face is living with someone who is aggressive and violent. Such problems can vary from acts of verbal abuse, through threats, to physical attacks of various intensities, with situations in which the relative's life is in danger at the extreme end. Estimates of violence in schizophrenic patients vary greatly, and a range of incidence between 8–45% of patients have been quoted. Although information booklets and other publicity frequently suggest that someone with schizophrenia is no more likely to be violent than any other member of the general population, this view has been challenged. Recent preliminary results from two on-going studies in the US (De Angelis, 1991) have reported opposite results. One study by Robert Zeiss and his colleagues found that schizophrenic patients who were judged to be a high risk for violent behaviour were more likely to fulfil this prediction than patients of other diagnoses. Another study by Edward Mulvey found that sufferers of schizophrenia were less likely to be dangerous than patients with other diagnoses.

A more pragmatic viewpoint for our purposes would be to examine under what conditions aggression and violence are more likely to occur, and what can be done to reduce the frequency and severity of such episodes. In the general population, violent acts are most likely to be committed by young males who have been drinking alcohol; with schizophrenic illness, episodes of aggression and violence may be more likely to be perpetrated by someone who is actively hallucinating or deluded; abuses drugs and alcohol; has been violent in the past either before they became ill or during illness episodes; has difficulties with anger control; or is experiencing high levels of tension.

Assessing the Determinants of Aggressive Behaviour

A behavioural analysis of aggressive acts is central to understanding how these can best be managed. Essentially, the procedures for conducting such an assessment follow the guidelines for assessing stressful situations (Chapter 6).

Firstly, an operational definition of what the relative means by an aggressive act is sought. What exactly does the patient do and say when he is being aggressive? Is there a range of behaviours, for example from shouting and swearing abuse at the relative or others, to damaging furniture or hitting people? If so, different categories of aggression should be agreed. For each category of behaviour, asking the relative to give a recent example is the best way to build up a picture of what factors may be precipitating and maintaining the behaviour. This picture includes:

1. What was happening before the aggressive behaviour occurred?
2. Was the relative (or others) aware that the patient was likely to become aggressive, and if so, when did they first notice signs of aggression, and what form did these take?
3. Did the relative try to do anything to prevent the aggressive behaviours occurring?
4. What exactly did the patient do and say, and how did others respond (thoughts, feelings, and behaviours)?
5. What were the outcomes for the patient, the relatives, and so on?

Having looked at one or two specific situations in some detail, the assessment can compare these to other situations when the patient is violent. Were the situations described typical? How were events similar/dissimilar to other situations? What makes things better/worse? We are looking here for patient factors such as mood, response to events and people, as well as relative factors, such as what the relative does and says.

Where possible, it is important to interview the patient and to attempt to obtain an analysis of the situations from them. Of particular importance is understanding how aware the patient is of the triggers, internal or external, of their aggression; what coping strategies, if any, they use to decrease their feelings of anger or other emotions associated with the aggression; and what are the consequences of the aggression for them in terms of feelings, behaviour, and thoughts. The use of record forms to monitor targeted situations at home will increase the accuracy of the relative's self-report, and will also allow you to evaluate progress once you begin an intervention programme.

The findings from the behavioural analysis will begin to shape intervention strategies, for example:

1. What factors are likely to increase the chance of the patient acting in an aggressive or violent manner?

2. Can these be changed?
3. Is the patient aware of the triggers for his/her aggressive behaviour?
4. What coping strategies does he/she have for dealing with angry feelings?
5. Could the patient learn to pay attention to triggers?
6. Could coping strategies be enhanced, or alternatives taught?
7. Is the reaction of the relative or others likely to escalate or defuse the aggression? Could the behavioural response of the relative or others be changed?
8. Does the threat of violence or the acts of verbal aggression have any function, for example, positive consequences, to the sufferer? For example, allowing a young man to get his own way with his mother, or as a means of coping with delusional thoughts or voices, and would it be possible to provide alternative ways of achieving this aim?

Case Examples

Bill has had schizophrenic symptoms since the age of 16. He was 18 at the time of the intervention. He lived with his mother, Jean, in a high-rise council flat, and neither was employed. He had frequent outbursts of temper directed at his mother, regularly kicked and damaged the furniture, had broken doors and windows, and had hit his mother on one recent occasion. His irritability ranged from daily periods of complaining to her, temper outbursts of verbal abuse about three times a week, to destructive episodes of throwing things or damaging the furniture about once a fortnight.

Bill's temper outbursts were targeted first for analysis. Signs of his irritability were apparent to his mother before the outbursts. These included complaints that his head felt tight, that life was not worth living, and his mother was not helping him. The immediate precipitant of an outburst was frequently a disagreement when Bill wanted his mother to do something, e.g., to give him some money, and his mother refused. Jean would then became frightened and anxious, lest Bill became violent. She would typically attempt to reason with him, explaining that there was insufficient money to give him any more, but often the situation developed into a two-way argument. His mother did not like to leave Bill alone during his aggressive periods lest he damaged himself or the flat, so she would sometimes withdraw to her bedroom. He would hammer on the door, and on one recent occasion had smashed the bedroom door down.

Bill was involved in the discussions as much as possible. He regretted his actions afterwards, but was unable to pinpoint the triggers of his irritability. Work was done to help him to try and identify the feelings associated with his irritability, and to find alternative ways of coping with these. The feelings were a tightness in his head and chest. A range of distracting activities was generated with him based on his interests, and included drawing, listening to music, and lying on his bed. During the intervention, Jean attempted to encourage Bill to use these alternatives when she observed his signs of irritability, and prompted him to label his feelings. When he began to challenge or criticize her behaviour, she offered him further reassurance and help with distraction, and would then withdraw from the house to visit a neighbour or friend. At the same time, Jean's needs for increased social interaction and activities away from Bill were targeted.

The interventions were successful in reducing the frequency and severity of the temper outbursts, and his mother established a daily break away from Bill.

Mr Gower had a four-year history of schizophrenia, and had persecutory delusions which he held with conviction, despite continued medication. He worked at a local factory and lived with his wife, who owned her own business. He was very suspicious of his workmates, and he believed his neighbours were spying on him. He frequently voiced his suspicions at home, becoming angry and calling them abusive names. On many occasions Mrs Gower would ignore her husband, but on the two or three evenings a week before she had to get up early to attend to her business she would have little patience, and would tell him to stop talking nonsense. Mr Gower would increase the intensity of his delusional ideas, and include his wife in a series of allegations and threats. The argument would then further intensify, with both parties losing their temper, shouting, and swearing at each other. Once every few months, either Mr or Mrs Gower would lose control and strike the other, who would then retaliate and a fight would ensue. These fights could be quite serious, with both parties receiving cuts and bruises. On one occasion Mr Gower had grabbed a carving knife from the kitchen table and chased his wife around the house until she had managed to lock herself in the bedroom. The fights would usually end with either the husband or wife taking refuge in the bedroom, or leaving the house.

It was clear from the analysis of the situations that arguments developed and physical fights occurred only when Mrs Gower challenged her husband's beliefs, and this usually happened if she wanted an early night and tried to shut him up. When she ignored his suspicions or even left the room, Mr Gower seemed to become calmer. Such strategies were discussed with the couple, and it was agreed that Mrs Gower would tell her husband that she disagreed with his suspicions, but that it was unhelpful to argue about them. If Mr Gower persisted and she was unable to ignore his rantings, she would leave the room, reminding him that this was part of their agreed plan.

The strategy was implemented with some success. There was a 50% decrease in the number of occasions when arguments occurred, and a significant reduction in Mr Gower's verbal abuse about the neighbours, although he retained full conviction that they were spying on him. This level of argument was acceptable to Mrs Gower, who may have inadvertently reinforced her husband's argumentative behaviour on some occasions. Since the onset of the illness, Mr Gower was much quieter, and showed little range of emotions. Mrs Gower felt it preferrable to retain some emotional reaction from her husband, albeit a negative one. Other interventions included advising Mrs Gower on managing her distress triggered by her husband's delusional talk, and coping with her feelings of loss since her husband had become withdrawn. Goal setting focused on increasing the range of enjoyable activities which the couple shared.

Where the Relative Over-Estimates the Likelihood of Violent Behaviour

In some cases relatives may grossly over-estimate the probability of both the occurrence and the severity of violent behaviour from the patient. Sometimes this may arise from an incident where the patient was violent towards objects or people as a consequence of delusional thinking, for example, they smashed up the TV set because they believed it was reading and transmitting their thoughts; or they attacked a person who they believed to be trying to kill them. When the psychotic symptoms have remitted, however, the likelihood of the patient behaving violently is very low. Or it may be that the relative is fearful that the patient may become violent, although there is no history of aggressive behaviour; or that verbal abuse or threats may lead to violence, but again there is no history of such occurrences.

Such relatives catastrophize the estimate of threat. One possible consequence is to avoid all possibilities of aggressive behaviours occurring, by, for example, always giving way to the patient's demands lest they become aggressive; or avoiding leaving them alone with other people lest arguments occur; or dissuading them from going out to pubs or social gatherings lest they get involved in fights. The relative may then attribute the fact that the feared aggressive behaviour never actually occurs to their avoidance of potential conflict situations, thereby reinforcing the relative's estimates of the success of their actions.

However, the relative may find there are major negative consequences of such strategies. Continually anticipating and fearing the worst may lead to considerable worry on their part; the strategy of avoiding conflict at all costs will likely lead to dissatisfactions and annoyance with the patient through continually giving way to their demands; and protecting them from external conflicts can result in reducing the patient's opportunities for independent functioning.

In these situations, there are two complementary approaches. Firstly, to deal with the relative's catastrophic estimates of the occurrence of violence. These over-estimates of threat can be dealt with using cognitive-behavioural methods (Chapter 6), which have been developed to deal with over-estimates of threat in anxiety patients (Hawton *et al.*, 1989; Blackburn and Davidson, 1990). The relatives' beliefs about the likelihood of the patient becoming violent or aggressive can be challenged through a combination of methods. For example, the relative can be encouraged to look at the evidence that the patient will become violent in the avoided situations, against the evidence that other outcomes are more likely. Often this approach will lead the relative to conclude that the likelihood of a violent reaction from the patient is actually very low, and the pros and cons of maintaining the avoidant actions can then be evaluated.

Secondly, where the fear of violence has led to the relative always giving way to the patient's demands, it will be necessary to help the relative to work out alternative ways of dealing with the demand situations: it is likely that some rehearsal of more assertive responses will be necessary, along with emotion-based coping strategies (Chapter 6). Following through the relative's worst possible fears may also help to decatastrophize their worries – 'What is the worst possible outcome you can imagine if you said no to his request?' – especially if you then work through a plan of action for the relative to take if the worst possible outcome happened.

Violent Behaviour

Although they represent a very small minority, some schizophrenic patients have a history of serious aggressive acts, and the risk of them committing serious violent assaults against relatives can be high. In the sample of patients studied in Salford, such patients were young, male, and residing in parental homes. The patients had persistent persecutory delusions, and had a history of alcohol or drug abuse.

Case Example

George was aged 32 and had been ill since his late teens, with persistent psychotic symptoms and a history of multiple hospital admissions. He lived with his retired parents, Mr and Mrs Brown, who were in their 70s. He had had a series of unskilled jobs in his teens, but had not been employed since then. For short periods he had lived away from home, but usually returned after a period of a few weeks.

While living at home, George would frequently go off for a few days and sometimes weeks on end without informing his parents of his whereabouts. He had been arrested by the police on a number of occasions for drunk and disorderly offences. At home, he spent much of the day in bed or listening to music, and there were frequent arguments between George and his father over his inactivity and the volume of the music.

During the past year, his mother reported that these arguments had become fiercer. Mrs Brown was physically frail and rarely left the house. During the weeks prior to George's most recent hospital admission, he had started to accuse Mr Brown that he was not in fact his father, and had physically attacked him on two occasions, the second resulting in a wound to his father's head, which required outpatient hospital treatment. Although they had contacted their GP and requested that George be admitted to hospital, it was only when George stabbed himself with a kitchen knife two weeks later that he was admitted to hospital. George committed a further assault on his father when on weekend leave from the ward, and his parents became increasingly fearful of his visits home.

After extensive discussions with George and his parents, it was decided that George be discharged from hospital to a hostel. After three months in hospital, he retained his delusions about his father with full conviction, and, given the history of conflict and violence, the risk of further assaults on his elderly father was assessed to be high. It was decided in agreement with all parties that George should visit his parents within prescribed times, with prior aggreement from his parents. Since George's violent attacks were usually only directed against his father, it was also agreed that his uncle, who lived close by, would also be in the house during George's visits. Lastly, it was agreed that if George turned up at the house outside of these 'visiting hours' or without prior warning, then his parents were not to let him in.

Unfortunately, George did frequently arrive at his parent's house outside of the negotiated times. On these occasions Mr and Mrs Brown stood by the agreed limits set on George's behaviour and refused him entry, although they found these situations very distressing. George was seen in the garden of his parent's house during the night, and on one occasion attempted to force entry into the house. When this happened Mr Brown called the police, which had been the agreed strategy. Because of the level of stress experienced by Mr and Mrs Brown in anticipating these visits at night, it was agreed that the staff at George's hostel should inform his parents if he went out very late at night or was away from the hostel overnight. As time went on George's visits to his parents decreased and were restricted to the prescribed times. There were no further assaults on the father, although George was sometimes verbally aggressive during his visits.

This case illustrates some of the difficulties in resolving family situations where the patient perpetrates repeated and serious agressive assaults against a family member. In all cases we experienced, the patient had a long illness history, and there is a possibility that earlier intervention may have improved the situation and resulted in a different outcome. In the case of George, apart from intermittent hospitalizations precipiated by acute crises, the family had little contact with mental health services. Interventions directed at improving the quality of George's independent functioning, help in resolving family conflicts, and possibly earlier settlement of George in alternative accommodation might have prevented the escalation of his aggressive behaviour towards his father.

SUICIDE

Although the risk of suicide is well recognized in depressive disorders, it has received much less attention in schizophrenia, even though it is a very real problem. Estimates of the suicide risk in sufferers of schizophrenia vary quite considerably. In an extensive review, Miles (1977) estimated that 10% of schizophrenia sufferers would die by suicide, although the rates reported in the different studies varied from 0.03% to 18%. A 40-year follow-up study (Tsuang, 1978) estimated the rates of suicide for sufferers of schizophrenia to be 4.1% overall, and 7% for men and 1% for women. In a recent review of suicides in schizophrenia by Caldwell and Gettesman (1990) a range, from the lowest of 1% for women to 12.5% for men was reported. Comparisons of suicide risk between schizophrenic patients and the normal population suggested that schizophrenic males were 21 times as likely to commit suicide as a general population of war veterans (Pokorny, 1983). Wilkinson (1982) estimated that a first admission schizophrenic patient was 56 to 83 times more likely to comit suicide than the person in the general population.

One of the variations are great and the methodologies and subject numbers different in these studies, it is clear that the risk for suicide in schizophrenia sufferers is markedly greater than in the general population, and approaches the risk for people suffering from major depressive disorders.

One of the essential elements in trying to prevent suicide is the identification of risk factors. Coldwell and Gettesman (1990) have outlined these known risk factors into two categories: personal risk factors that are common to both the general population and schizophrenia sufferers; and risk factors that appear specific to schizophrenia patients:

Risk Factors Common to Both the General Population and Schizophrenia

- depression or depressed mood
- sense of hopelessness
- past history of suicide attempts
- family history of suicide
- unmarried
- unemployed
- deteriorating health with high levels of premorbid functioning
- recent loss or rejection
- parental loss during childhood
- limited external support
- family stress and instability

Risk Factors Specific to Schizophrenia

- young and male
- chronic illness with numerous exacerbations
- high levels of psychopathology and functional impairment following discharge
- realistic awareness of deteriorating effects of the illness and a non-delusional negative assessment of the future
- fear of further mental deterioration
- excessive treatment dependence and/or loss of faith in treatment.

From these risk factors it would appear that a classical risk profile would be of a young, unmarried, and unemployed male, who experiences increasingly frequent acute exacerbations, with residual symptoms and disabilities between episodes. He would typically have had a good pre-morbid personality with reasonable aspirations for the future. During periods of insight he would probably feel his future now holds little for him other than a deteriorating illness and further mental anguish, which treatment will fail to abate. He will probably have a history of suicide attempts, be socially isolated, and have restricted access to social support.

In the general population, factors such as impulsivity, aggressivity, frustration intolerance, alcohol abuse, and the use of more lethal means of self-injury are associated with men taking their lives more frequently than women. These factors also increase the risk in male sufferers of schizophrenia. However, schizophrenia appears to reduce the inhibitions to suicide usually found in women.

Assessment of Suicide Risk

Sufferers of schizophrenia who have a large number of these risk factors are likely to be a continuing and long-term suicide risk. A good relationship with the patient will help the therapist to evaluate whether this risk is increasing over the short-term. Evidence that the patient is unusually depressed, hopeless or pessimistic about the future should be taken seriously. Risk appears to increase soon after the patient is discharged from hospital, or soon after the psychotic symptoms remit. This may be because the patient has developed sufficient insight to develop a pessimistic view about the future, especially if they had high aspirations before they became ill.

If there is evidence of depressed mood or hopelessness, the therapist should attempt to elicit whether the patient has had ideas of harming or killing themselves. If so, the therapist should determine whether they have any plans about how they would do so, and if they have made any preparations to carry out these plans, such as by storing pills or obtaining a firearm or poison. The therapist should also ascertain whether the usual constraints and inhibitions to suicide are breaking down, such as the loss to friends and family, duties and obligations, especially to family and children, and religious or cultural mores; many of these inhibitions to suicide may not be operative in the high-risk group anyway. Furthermore, whether there have been any precipitators or crises, especially involving rejection or highlighting the disabilities associated with suffering from schizophrenia.

The presence of many of these factors would clearly indicate an increase in risk. However, although patients who are severely psychotic do commit suicide, suicide attempts in response to symptoms are reported to be rare (Caldwell and Gettesman, 1990). However, they do occur, and in response to a variety of delusional thinking. For example, in our study, one young man made two serious attempts on his life because of persecutory beliefs; while another attempted to commit suicide because he was convinced a member of the Royal Family was inhabiting his body, and it was therefore his duty, as a gentleman, to vacate it.

HELPING RELATIVES TO COPE WITH THE RISK OF SUICIDE

Although the occurrence of suicide is greatly inflated in sufferers of schizophrenia compared to that of the general population, there are also occasions when patients may frequently threaten suicide but the risk of death is low. The problems here are how to assess actual suicide risk, and how to cope with threats or fears of suicide when the probability of the patient seriously injuring or killing themself is low. The following case examples should help to emphasize these difficulties.

Case Example

Alex was a 22-year-old man who lived with his divorced mother. He had been ill for approximately three years, and reported persistent symptoms of delusions and auditory hallucinations. His level of functioning was very low, he hardly ever left the house, and he spent most of the time lying on his bed or the settee, or occasionally watching television. He had a close and supportive relationship with his mother, and would frequently seek reassurance from her about his preoccupations with his belief that he had brain damage, and his voices.

Alex monopolized much of his mother's attention, and since he disliked leaving the house or being left alone, she spent most of the time at home. She had given up her job to care for him, felt herself to blame for his illness, and had become estranged from other members of her family, including an older son and daughter, because of her devotion to Alex.

Alex had made at least twelve attempts at suicide, including one occasion when he had attempted to hang himself from the stairwell while his mother was speaking on the telephone to her sister. He frequently alluded to the fact that his life was not worth living, and that he might as well be dead. Such ideas made his mother very distressed, and she felt he needed her continued presence to help him to cope with his depressed moods, and she was fearful of leaving him in the house alone.

The intervention followed the guidelines for the management of stressful and difficult situations outlined in Chapter 6. An analysis of the situations when Alex reported distress and sought reassurance from his mother helped her to see that the consequences of giving Alex repeated reassurance, although helpful to Alex in the short term, had considerable negative consequences for herself and for him in the longer term. Unfortunately, Alex was not happy to co-operate with plans to change the pattern of interactions in the home, so it was not possible to work with him on increasing his range of independent strategies to cope with his symptoms; he also refused to attend a local day centre.

Given that Alex was reluctant to co-operate with the plans, his mother required a great deal of support to try out alternative ways of responding to his comfort requests. Work was done on helping her to make a realistic assessment of the risks of withdrawing some of her support, before she began a carefully graded programme of spending increasingly longer periods away from the home, which she spent visiting other members of her family.

The interventions had some limited success in reducing the mother's belief that Alex's well-being and safety from self-harm was dependent on the level of reassurance she gave him. Although Alex was at first unhappy with his mother leaving the house, he later agreed to participate in working at some small goals for increasing his self-care skills within the home. This provided his mother with the opportunity for increasing the amount of attention she gave him for purposeful activities within the home.

Case Example

The second case is somewhat different and has a less happy outcome. John had a six-year history of schizophrenia and had lived with his parents throughout this time. Over the course of the intervention his parents had been very successful in learning appropriate ways of coping both with their own distress and with John's illness. John had moved into a flat of his own and had held a part-time job for over a year. It was 18 months since his last relapse, during which time he had been free of schizophrenic symptoms. John usually saw his parents once every one to two weeks, and everything appeared to be going well. He also saw his married sister regularly, but she and her husband has been having marital problems and had split up the previous week. John had stayed at his parents' house on the Sunday night, and returned to his flat on the Monday morning so as to go to work in the afternoon. He had made some lunch for himself, but without touching it he had gone out of his flat and thrown himself from a close-by motorway bridge. He was killed instantly.

John's suicide seemed to occur out of the blue. Although he had many of the previously listed risk factors, he had made considerable improvements in his level of social and independent functioning, and his quality of life had objectively improved from earlier in his illness. Perhaps this was the very problem: although John had improved and the family were extremely happy with his progress, these gains had overshadowed the continuing high risk of suicide. John had made considerable progress from when he had been living at home and been highly dependent on his parents. At the time of his death he had a much more relaxed relationship with his parents, a part-time job, and a flat of his own. These were all things he had targeted as long-term goals when the family intervention had first started. However, John was still lonely and had few friends, none of which could have been described as providing a confiding relationship.

Two other factors can be considered important: firstly, access to his one strong relationship outside of his parents – his sister – had recently been greatly restricted because of her own marital difficulties. Secondly, his mother had severe health problems of her own, and was subsequently diagnosed as suffering from breast cancer, although this was not known at the time of John's death. But John was aware of his mother's ill health and his father's concern.

These two life events needed to be considered in the context of John's desire not to be a burden upon his family, and his increasing realization that although benefits were being achieved from treatment, these improvements would be marginal compared to what he had once hoped for in his life. In these circumstances, John's suicide was probably neither impulsive – although the actual timing of it may have been – nor unpredictable.

It is important to continually review the circumstances of patients who have the risk characteristics for suicide. Furthermore, attention to details of life changes such as loss or rejection, which may further isolate the patient is crucial; and improvements in their social functioning may indicate an increased, rather than decreased, risk for suicide. Care needs to be taken that intensive interventions are not suddenly curtailed, withdrawing social supports and, in some cases, a sense of optimism for further improvement. In these cases it is important that alternative social support systems are made available either through the mental health services, if appropriate, or through other non-professional alternatives.

Chapter 10

Other Psychological Methods Useful in the Management of Schizophrenia

Over the past few years there has been a growing interest in the use of psychological methods of management as adjuncts to pharmacological management. Besides family intervention methods, a number of other areas of management are potentially useful. The two areas that have received the most attention are the use of psychological methods to control residual psychotic symptoms, and the use of early-signs monitoring to identify imminent relapse. For the professional who is setting up a family intervention programme, some knowledge of these other methods may be useful. One possibility would be to integrate all of them into an overall service for patients suffering from schizophrenia.

PSYCHOLOGICAL MANAGEMENT OF POSITIVE SCHIZOPHRENIC SYMPTOMS

Studies carried out with patients living in the community, and with those living in long-stay services in psychiatric hospitals have shown that a considerable number of patients continue to experience positive psychotic symptoms. Estimates are that 40–50% of such groups still exhibit hallucination or delusions, even with aggressive medication (Silverstein *et al.*, 1978; Curson *et al.*, 1985; 1988). These residual symptoms may not be as intense or as pervasive compared to those that occurred during the acute episode, but they appear to be chronic in nature and resistant to further improvement with pharmacological treatment. Furthermore, the experience of these continued symptoms can be extremely distressing, can increase the possibility of suicide, and severely disrupt the level of functioning of the patient (Falloon, 1986).

Various psychological methods have been utilized successfully to alleviate such symptoms, including the application of rewards and punishments; self-instruction; stimulus control; belief modification; thought stopping; the manipulation of auditory stimulation; and self-control (Hemsley, 1986; Heinrichs, 1988; Slade *et al.*, 1988; Tarrier, 1991c; 1991d). These reports have usually been case studies or small uncontrolled studies applied in a wide variety of settings with different patient groups. Few controlled trials have been carried out, and there is little information about how generally these findings could apply.

Other studies have indicated that many patients attempt to use psychological or behavioural methods to cope with their symptoms (Falloon *et al.*, 1981; Breier *et al.*, 1983; Tarrier, 1987). Since coping methods are used naturally by many patients, attempting to systematically instruct patients how to cope with their symptoms has a number of attractions as a method of psychological management.

Coping methods may be aimed at reducing the symptoms themselves, or reducing the emotional reaction they cause – or both of these. It is assumed that although some symptoms may occur endogenously, many symptoms will arise in response to specific precipitators. These may be environmental events and situations, such as social interaction or periods of inactivity, or they may be internal events such as specific thought patterns or high levels of arousal. Endogenous or biological factors may result in the occurrence of psychotic symptoms through some common pathway such as the arousal system. It is further assumed that the presence of symptoms such as hallucinations and delusions will have specific consequences for the patient: initially an emotional reaction such as anxiety or anger; short-term consequences such as social disengagement and general avoidance; and also more long-term consequences, such as restricted social interactions as the patient attempts to limit the aversive nature of both the symptoms and the emotional reaction that they evoke.

Since the emotional response to experiencing a delusion or hallucination may also create the conditions in which more hallucinations and delusions are experienced by resulting in higher levels of arousal, the symptoms and the emotions they produce are potentially linked in a downward negative spiral. The increasing frequency of psychotic symptoms and negative emotions may also increase the contact the patient has with the environment that brought about the symptoms in the first place.

The environmental cues, the experience of the psychotic symptoms, their emotional consequences, and their medium- and long-term effects are all linked in a complex manner which has a negative impact on the sufferer's life. A diagramatic representation of the interaction of these factors is presented in Figure 10.1.

The aim of treatment is to break into this negative spiral and reverse the process. If the symptoms themselves cannot be reduced, then their emotional impact can be alleviated; however, it is also possible that in reducing their negative consequences, the symptoms will decrease.

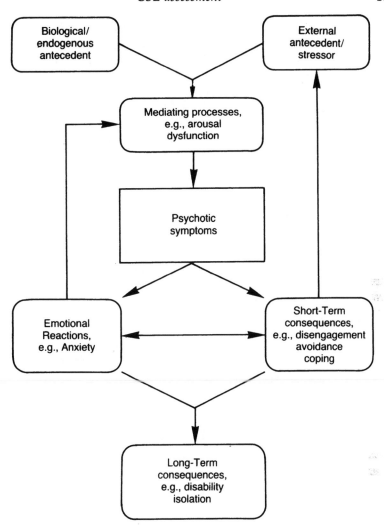

Figure 10.1 Heuristic Model of Psychotic Symptoms.

This method of psychological treatment aims to teach patients methods of coping with their symptoms. Where possible, the goal is to enhance coping strategies already being used by the patient, and so the procedure has been termed Coping Strategy Enhancement (CSE).

CSE ASSESSMENT

Central to CSE is an assessment procedure to examine the specific and idiosyncratic relationships between environmental context, psychotic symptoms, and their consequences in a particular individual. The assessment interview should follow a collaborative problem-solving approach, in which the patient and the clinician work together to find out more details about the patient's experience.

It is necessary to give the patient a detailed rationale for this exercise. If the patient is convinced that his or her delusions or hallucinations are real, and does not agree that these experiences are in anyway illness related, then the focus of the rationale for the intervention can be directed towards reducing the distress and upset these experiences cause.

Format for the Assessment Interview

Type of Symptom

Define and describe each of the psychotic symptoms the patient experiences. The Present State Examination glossary (Wing *et al.*, 1974), and the BPRS seven-point rating scale for hallucinations and unusual thought content (Lukoff *et al.*, 1986) are useful for defining and rating symptoms.

Nature of Symptoms

For each of the symptoms so described, ascertain the frequency, duration, and intensity of their occurrence. This becomes more difficult when the symptoms are less circumscribed and do not have clearly identifiable onset and offset points. If there are variations, try to obtain the common occurrence and an estimate of the range of what can occur. The patient can be asked to self-monitor their symptoms to help clarify this information, which may also help the patient to become more aware of their symptoms, and to distinguish them from normal experience.

Antecedents

For each symptom, elicit the situations in which that symptom occurs, looking for situations or common characteristics of situations in which each symptom is more likely to occur. It is possible that symptoms will appear to occur at random, but also cluster with higher frequency in some situations. For example, symptoms may be more likely to occur when the patient is inactive, or when they are in specific social situations. The experience of symptoms that occur 'out of the blue' can be thought of as endogenous – occurring at any time, possibly due to some biological process – and those that appear to be situational can be thought of as reactive – being situation-specific because of an interaction between an environmental context and a biological process. Initially, external environmental situations should be asked about, and when these possibilities have been exhausted, then those internal events – thoughts, images, and physical sensations – should be covered.

This part of the interview should provide as comprehensive a picture of the antecedents and precipitating conditions as possible. Self-monitoring can also be used for clarification.

Emotional Reactions

For each symptom, the immediate emotional consequence should be elicited. This should be described in terms of how it makes the patient feel (physical sensations); what sort of thoughts and cognitions they have; and, if appropriate, the effect on their behaviour. This is best achieved by first asking general and open-ended questions concerning the emotional reactions, and second, having identified these as occurring, to ask more specific questions.

Consequences

For each symptom, the more long-term consequences should be elicited. That is, what happens in response to the emotional reaction, usually in terms of the patient's behaviour, for example, what they did next, such as avoiding going out, or shouting at the voices, or any other actions.

Methods of Coping

Elicit whether the patient does anything to cope with each symptom or the emotions associated with it. Coping implies an active attempt to master, control, or overcome the symptom or the distress it causes. Coping should not be confused with the consequences of the symptom, although there will be some overlap, such as when the patient withdraws from social interactions. Coping should refer to an overt or covert action, which is carried out with the intention of producing a positive or appropriate outcome.

Having elicited any coping strategies used by the patient, their effectiveness can be rated simply by using a three-point scale where zero equals no or little effect; one equals minor or temporary improvement; and two equals major and long-lasting improvement.

This assessment process may take some time, and many psychotic patients may be intolerant of long periods of social interaction. In such cases, the assessment should take place over a number of sessions tailored to the patient's individual capabilities. If the patient does appear stressed at any point, it may be worth questioning them about any intensification of their symptoms happening at that time. Clinical judgement should be exercised carefully, however, so as not to stress the patient further – it is best to err on the side of caution.

COPING STRATEGIES

Past research has indicated that it is possible to categorize different methods of coping (Tarrier, 1987). Although these divisions can be somewhat arbitrary, they serve a practical function of helping the clinician think in detail about the appropriate coping methods to teach the patient.

Cognitive Strategies

These strategies attempt to control the symptoms by a change in cognitive or thought processes.

Attention-Switching

Here, the patient switches their attention from one subject to another, as in focusing attention on distracting thoughts. It assumes that the capacity of immediate attention is limited, so that an active switching from one subject to another will decrease the probability of the former remaining in attention. This might include, for example, teaching the patient to concentrate on a positive and reinforcing image such as a tropical beach or a pleasant holiday when they experience a delusional thought or an hallucination. This appears to be a common and effective coping method.

Attention-Narrowing

This occurs when attention is restricted, or when a subject is excluded from attention without being replaced. Examples of attention-narrowing are thought-stopping, or when the patient clears their mind or blanks out their thoughts. This strategy can be useful in the short term, but in the long term it is very difficult not to think of a subject or to think of nothing without refocusing attention.

Self-Instruction

Here the patient instructs themselves or engages in a covert dialogue either to assess a situation or to cue behaviour. Such covert verbal behaviour can be very effective in both relabelling illness-related experiences and in prompting positive coping strategies. Such as: 'The voices aren't real, they cannot hurt me, they're just part of the illness' and 'I must concentrate on relaxing and slowing my breathing.'

Rational Restructuring

This refers to a complex set of psychological processes by which the experience of the psychotic symptoms are tested in reality. The procedure of 'reality testing' may include behavioural elements, but the evaluative process is psychological. This process involves the generation of alternative hypotheses to 'prove' the symptom to be 'real' or illness-related. Evidence to support or refute these hypotheses is then collected and evaluated. There is reason to believe this method works well with some patients, however, with those who have either no insight or complete conviction in the reality of their symptoms, difficulty can arise. With the latter group, it may be possible to first weaken the strength of the belief in the symptom by the use of other coping strategies.

Behavioural Strategies

These attempt to control symptoms by a change in overt action.

Engaging in Solitary Activities

Here, the patient engages in an activity in response to their symptom that does not involve others. This could include: going for a walk alone, reading, exercise, making something, etc. This strategy involves some element of distraction, and is frequently used to decrease the patient's level of arousal.

Social Withdrawal

This involves actively disengaging from social contact. It is effectively an escape or avoidance response, and can have severe long-term consequences in terms of social isolation. Undeniably, many patients find prolonged social interactions highly stressful, hence the stress-reducing and reinforcing value associated with escape from and avoidance of social contact.

As a coping strategy withdrawal can be used, but should be used carefully. Patients should be encouraged to use disengagement as a means of gradually building up tolerance to social situations and as a temporary stress-reduction technique. That is, they should be set goals of gradually increasing their length of tolerance of social situations before disengaging. Disengagement should then be used as a rest period during which arousal levels decrease before the patient re-enters the social interaction. Patients should be encouraged to functionally disengage rather than physically disengage. This would mean, for example, withdrawing from the conversation rather than leaving the room.

Engaging in Social Interaction

A surprising number of patients report that engaging in social interaction is an effective coping strategy. A further attribute of this method is that it normalizes the patient's level of functioning, and it can be socially appropriate. Presumably, overt conversation helps to interrupt and inhibit internal events such as psychotic symptoms.

Physiological Strategies

These strategies attempt to control the symptoms by producing a change in the patient's physiological state.

Relaxation and/or Breathing Exercises

Physiological strategies such as the various methods of relaxation – progressive muscle relaxation, autogenic relaxation, differential relaxation or breathing exercises – can be extremely helpful in both de-arousing and distracting the patient. Performing such exercises can break the chain of symptom, events between emotional distress, and psychotic behaviour. Besides potentially decreasing the anxiety accompanying such symptoms, there is the possibility of decreasing the symptoms themselves by decreasing the level of arousal that precipitates them. (These methods are used commonly in the behavioural treatments of anxiety, but with this patient population extra care should be taken, and extended practice should be given.)

Pharmacological Agents and Alcohol

Patients will often attempt to self-medicate themselves by abusing alcohol, street drugs, and prescription drugs. Clearly these methods should not be encouraged, however, it is probably unrealistic to expect patients to stop their habits once they have become established. If this is the case, then moderation should be aimed for with the augmentation of alternative methods of stress reduction, such as relaxation. The reasonable use of alcohol in appropriate social settings, such as a pub, would seem to be socially normative.

Sensory Strategies

These strategies use the change in sensory input to control symptoms. Such methods as listening to the radio or a personal stereo or using ear plugs have been tried with varying degrees of success. Attention should be paid to the social appropriateness of the method used. It may also be possible to pair other techniques, such as self-instruction, with modifications of sensory input. Self-instruction would then be reinforced as a coping method as it would be associated with symptom reduction, and the use of sensory modification could then be phased out (see the case example below).

TEACHING COPING STRATEGIES

From the above descriptions, it is apparent that a wide range of coping strategies are available to the clinician. There are a number of guidelines that can help in their implementation.

1. First, work on building and strengthening coping strategies that are already in use. These are termed entry strategies since they allow entry into a new mode of functioning.
2. Break down each strategy into its basic components, teach each component separately as a technique, and finally increase the size of the teaching unit by combining the techniques.
3. Practise extensively, and never assume the patient knows how to perform a coping strategy; practise until the strategy becomes overlearnt and can be performed automatically. This will greatly increase the chances of it being performed in vivo.
4. If possible, practise the coping strategies when the symptoms actually occur. If they do not occur during the treatment session, then attempt to simulate them. For example, the therapist can verbalize the delusional thought out loud so that the patient can use strategies to cope with it. A similar procedure can be used with hallucinations.
5. In teaching cognitive coping strategies, start the procedure with overt verbalizations and slowly fade into covert verbalizations. Similarly, commence with the overt verbalizations coming from the therapist, and then introduce the patient into making overt verbalizations of the appropriate coping strategy. Finally, these overt verbalizations are practiced covertly by the patient. For example if a distracting image is to be used, then this should be described out loud, first by the therapist and then by the patient. The patient should then attempt a covert description and image.
6. Arrange contingencies to reinforce positive coping. Coping should have a positive consequence, such as the reduction in anxiety and the elicitation of social reinforcement from the therapist. If the reduction in the frequency of the symptom results in the patient becoming unoccupied or bored, make sure alternative activities are included in the treatment programme.

7. Select one symptom to treat first and focus on it until marked improvement is obtained. If success is not immediately achieved, maintain the effort. It is not advisable to jump from symptom to symptom.
8. Select the first symptom to be treated on the basis of the greatest chance of success. For example, the patient has already established coping strategies which can be further enhanced, except when a symptom causes severe distress or disruption, in which case, address this one first.
9. While patients should be encouraged to monitor and record their symptoms, focusing on the occurrence of symptoms can be counterproductive; if possible select a variable to be recorded that is indicative of improvement or absence of symptoms.

Case Example

Mrs Eddy, a 58-year-old woman, had first been diagnosed as suffering from schizophrenia when she was 25. She had had only five admissions to hospital, the last being one being 18 months previously, but had continued to experience psychotic symptoms of one degree or another throughout her illness. She had not worked since first becoming ill, and had lived a fairly restricted life. She lived with her husband, but had little contact with him as he worked long hours and had distanced himself emotionally from her because of her illness. She now spent most of her day alone, although she received some support from her neighbours. Mrs Eddy was able to care for herself, but only left the house rarely. She went to the local village for her shopping, and attended a local church social group twice a week, and the church service on Sundays.

Mrs Eddy experienced auditory hallucinations at least once a day for up to two to three hours, in which she heard at least two or three voices discussing her in an obscene and hostile manner. She frequently thought the voices were local people hiding outside her house. Because of her sheltered life and religious views, these hallucinations caused her intense distress. In the company of other people she frequently felt they knew what she was thinking because they could hear her thoughts. She believed that everybody thought she was a disgusting person. She experienced delusions of reference and misinterpretation, since certain signs such as traffic-light changes and the angle of parked cars indicated what a shameful person she was.

Usually Mrs Eddy felt relaxed at her church social group since she knew the people well, however, on one occasion as she was leaving the church hall she experienced auditory hallucinations saying obscene and blasphamous phrases. She became very upset because she believed her friends also heard the voices, and, thinking it was her saying these things, they were disgusted with her. On the following day, she saw one of the members of the church social group drive past her in a car while she had been out shopping. Because her friend had not acknowledged her, she was further convinced the women at the social group had rejected her. Mrs Eddy stopped attending the church altogether, became increasingly distressed, and the psychotic symptoms became more frequent. The only way she could control the voices was to drown them out by turning on the vacuum cleaner.

Intervention

Initially, Mrs Eddy was taught to identify the voices as being illness related. When she heard them, she was instructed to say to herself, 'The voices are part of my illness; they're not real; they cannot hurt me.' She experienced great difficulty in managing this unless the intensity of the hallucinations was reduced by the noise of the vacuum cleaner. Constant use of the vacuum cleaner to drown out the hallucinations was clearly not appropriate, so she substituted the radio, which she had previously never listened to.

Mrs Eddy was also taught breathing and autogenic relaxation exercises, so that the onset of the hallucinations could be a cue to physically relax and repeat the positive statements. Relaxation also served as a distraction, and was used as an alternative to switching on the radio. Her ability to relax also served to reduce her levels of distress. As her levels of tension decreased, Mrs Eddy's ability to concentrate increased, and she was able to further distract herself once she had relaxed by reading. With practice she could relabel the voices as part of her illness, relax, and engage herself in reading. The frequency, intensity, and duration of the hallucinations diminished, and her mood and confidence greatly improved.

The incident at her church social group was discussed. It was suggested that if the hallucinations and delusions of reference were part of the illness, then the other members of the group would not have heard the voices, nor would they hold negative opinions about her, and would most probably welcome her back to the group. If, however, her interpretation of the events were true, then the group would most probably not welcome her back. If the group did reject her, she had not really lost anything since she believed this to have happened anyway, whereas, if she had been wrong, she had everything to gain.

Mrs Eddy agreed to put these two alternative hypotheses to the test by attending the next social group meeting. Although she was not optimistic of the outcome, she felt confident enough to attempt the task because she felt so much better at home. She attended the meeting, and was surprised to find that all her friends were pleased to see her, and there was no mention of the obscene voices.

At the next treatment session, Mrs Eddy agreed that all her psychotic experiences were due to her illness, although they had seemed real. Interestingly, this rational interpretation reversed over the next month. When asked about the event she said she was convinced the voices had been heard by her friends, but clearly they had forgiven her since the topic was never spoken about. This interpretation proved beneficial since although she occasionally experienced psychotic phenomena, they caused her little concern since no one else seemed bothered by them either.

Mrs Eddy's husband played a minimal role, being encouraged to praise her achievements and to ignore any psychopathology. This was the most he was prepared to contribute to the intervention, and, in this case, it was probably appropriate. In other cases, relatives could be used more extensively, such as to prompt patients in the use of their coping strategies and to systematically reinforce their use; to assist patients in reality testing; and to engage patients in activities in cases where inactivity is an antecedent to symptoms.

PRODROMAL SIGNS AND EARLY INTERVENTION

There is now reasonable evidence to suggest that many sufferers of schizophrenia experience a characteristic prodromal phase before relapsing (Herz *et al.*, 1980; Subotnik *et al.*, 1988; Birchwood *et al.*, 1989, 1991). Typically, this prodromal phase lasts from a few days to about four weeks, during which clusters of neurotic symptoms begin to appear and intensify in the period leading up to relapse. In some patients, there is also an increase in psychotic or unusual experiences which lead into a full-blown relapse. Some authors (Doherty *et al.*, 1978) indicate there are two phases within the prodromal period: an initial phase characterized by an increase in neurotic symptoms, and a second phase in which increases in psychotic symptoms predominate. However, opinions on this biphasic nature of the prodromal period vary.

It does appear that patients have a characteristic prodromal period before relapse, which has been aptly labelled the patient's 'relapse signature' by Birchwood and his colleagues. This relapse signature represents a pattern of prodromal signs and symptoms which are idiosyncratic to the patient and herald imminent relapse. They are frequently recognized as such by both the patient and those who know him or her well. In fact, relatives frequently complain they can recognize when the patient is about to relapse but are unable to obtain help from the mental health services at that point, even though a full relapse could be avoided.

Table 10.2 Signs and Symptoms Reported as Present During the Prodromal Period of Schizophrenic Relapse

Tense and nervous	Ideas of reference
Afraid and anxious	Increase in religious thinking
Trouble sleeping	Hears voices or sees things
Depressed	Behaves as though hallucinating
Low	Beliefs of external control
Quiet and withdrawn	Odd behaviour
Eating less and poor appetite	Feeling suspicious or puzzled
Loss of weight	Fears of going mad
Trouble concentrating	Talking in an incoherent way
Enjoying things less	
Preoccupied	
Cannot remember things	
Seeing friends less	
Loss of interest	
Feeling bad for no reason	
Feeling worthless	
Loss of interest in appearance	
Thoughts of hurting or killing self	
Frequent aches and pains	
Restlessness	
Violent and/or aggressive	
Stubborn	
Feeling excited	
Bad dreams	
Feeling angry at minor irritations	
Difficulty with partner	
Increase in abuse of drugs or alcohol	

(Adapted from Herz *et al.*, 1980; Birchwood *et al.*, 1989).

The array of typical signs and symptoms that have been described in the literature are indicated in Table 10.2.

The idea that an imminent relapse could be identified and some intervention applied to abort it is an appealing one which has received some empirical support (Herz *et al.*, 1991). Such preventative measures would also receive much support from relatives, who frequently feel the frustration of the services only reacting in response to crisis rather than to avoid one. Patients would also, in the main, prefer not to experience a full-blown relapse and all its consequences, such as social disruption and hospitalization. Most of the research suggests that insight is retained through the prodromal period, and in many cases up until the day of relapse, indicating that early intervention may be both possible and welcomed. The possibility of accurately being able to identify imminent relapse opens up a number of possibilities for innovative management.

Close collaboration between the services, patient, and their family means that prodromes could be identified and preventative measures implemented so as to abort relapse. The exact nature of these preventative measures and their optimum implementation has yet to be determined. Clearly, pharmacological intervention is likely to be effective and efficient and has much to recommend it. Psychosocial management such as a family management and symptom management have considerable appeal, but are as yet untested in these circumstances. However, there is no reason why such preventative strategies should not be incorporated into a psychosocial management plan.

Neuroleptic medication used over long periods of time has many disadvantages, but if imminent relapse could be identified it may be possible to withdraw suitable patients from prophylactic medication and use medication in an intermittent and targeted manner when prodromal signs become apparent. Quite a lot has been written about intermittent and targeted medication strategies and the use of 'drug holidays' (Carpenter and Heinrichs, 1983; Heinrichs *et al.*, 1985; Jolley *et al.*, 1989; Herz *et al.*, 1991) and there is considerable appeal to these methods, under the correct circumstances. To function well, close liaison between the patient, their family, and professionals would be required, and the resources within the mental health services to provide the necessary monitoring and response capability.

Many patients refuse to take their medication or poorly comply with their treatment. They are usually thought of as difficult, and are unpopular with staff because of their excessive use of resources. The services are also unpopular with these patients, who frequently perceive them as restricting their freedom. This situation is clearly not going to be resolved by some sort of battle of will between these 'difficult' patients and the mental health services. Better to reach some kind of compromise, for example, if this group of patients could be taught to identify their relapse signatures and agreed to seek help when these occurred, and the services agreed to provide the appropriate assistance when the patient identified they needed it, then some movement towards a solution of how to meet the needs of this population may be possible.

SUMMARY

In summary, although the work on prodromal signs and early intervention is in its infancy, it is exciting because of the number of options it opens up. Similarly, the use of psychological management methods with patients who experience residual psychotic symptoms also increases the number of intervention strategies open to the clinician. Clearly not all patients will benefit, and as yet we are unable to suggest what are predictors of good outcome for psychological management. It is important not to view family interventions as the only option available, particularly when family members refuse to participate, or when the family is cynical about the prospect of changing or improving the patient and are reluctant to collaborate with the therapist to that end; or when the patient's symptoms are so severe it is difficult for families to work directly with the patient to co-operate in plans for change.

It should also be remembered that other well-established intervention strategies, such as social skills training and life skills training, may also be appropriately and effectively used. The therapist should keep in mind as many options as possible to augment and facilitate family interventions.

Chapter 11

Working Within Service Organizations

Health care professionals who intend to introduce family intervention programmes will probably be working as part of an organization. Usually, although not necessarily, this is a public health service.

The introduction of a new service requires new ways of working and organizational change, producing change within the organization so that the new service can be implemented and developed can be problematic. Although one might expect that a new intervention method would be easy to implement, since it will improve the current practice of the service, this is rarely the case. Georgiades and Phillimore (1975), in their article on producing organizational change, call this 'the myth of the hero-innovator'. They make the analogy of a knight errant, who, armed with new interventions, treatment strategies, and beliefs intends to assault the 'organizational fortress and institute change, both in himself and others, at a stroke'. The reality is somewhat different. As Georgiades and Phillimore say, 'organizations such as . . . hospitals, like dragons, eat hero-innovators for breakfast.'

To produce new services means changing the behaviour of other staff, probably at all levels. Change can be difficult to produce, and very difficult to sustain. Organizations tend to have a homeostatic process of inertia, and it can be very difficult and frustrating for an enthusiastic clinician wanting to start a new service to come up against such inertia.

This chapter outlines some of the issues and difficulties staff may encounter, and some possible solutions. We do this in two ways: firstly, to summarize the guidance outlined by Georgiades and Phillimore on how to 'ensure that such organizations receive newly trained hero-innovators without gobbling them up'; and, secondly, by recounting some of our own experiences and some of the issues we became aware of while managing the Salford Project.

LESSONS FROM GEORGIADES AND PHILLIMORE'S GUIDELINE ON ORGANIZATIONAL CHANGE

In order to bring about change that will benefit clients, it may be necessary to move away from a one-to-one treatment relationship into the role of an organizational change agent or a manager of change. In terms of family intervention, this means attention has to be paid to preparing the organizational culture in which the family intervention will be implemented. A second and related point is that since organizational change is a slow process – estimates of three to five years are given for change within commercial or industrial organizations – it will probably be necessary to review the time course of the development of new services, which relates to the earlier point made about the homeostasis of inertia. Developing a family intervention programme without first preparing the groundwork for organizational change may result in the new service being short-lived; to achieve permanent change, time and adequate preparation are required.

These two points emphasize the necessity of 'cultivating the host culture'. There are a number of ways this can be accomplished, depending on the available resources. It is desirable to have a nominated person, preferably quite senior, to be the organizational change manager, who is responsible for preparing and cultivating the service host culture so it is receptive to the required change. The organizational change manager may delegate responsibilities where appropriate, but they should be responsible for determining the overall strategic plan of implementing the new service through facilitating the organizational process.

Overall Strategies

There are two overall strategies: first, to maximize the impact of the scarce resources available by exerting influence through strengths and expertise; and second, to instil and maintain a team identity for the group involved in the family intervention service.

The maintenance of high morale within the team, especially when difficulties and stresses are confronted, is not just important but essential to the success of the endeavour. Team cohesion and morale can be maintained through, for example: keeping the team to manageable numbers; maintaining regular contact between team members; involving all team members in decision-making; and updating team members on the progress of the project.

In the Salford Project, we found that weekly meetings that included everyone involved with the Project were useful in maintaining a cohesive team. The meetings involved updating the clinical and administrative staff with details of all of the families in the Project, and an action plan of who was to do what, and when, with whom. The action plan was operationalized in the minutes of the meeting, and reviewed at subsequent meetings. Besides acting as a case review of all assessment and treatment plans for each family in the Project, the meetings also informed team members of progress, and allowed them to problem-solve any difficulties. This type of case review/progress report meeting is recommended for all teams involved in family intervention programmes.

Specific Strategies

'The organizational change manager should work with the people within the organization who are positive and supportive rather than against those who are negative or defensive.'

It is appropriate to use psychological skills and sensitivity to uncover the determinants of facilitation, or resistance to implementation, of a family intervention programme, be they personal or organizational. It is necessary to know under what conditions people would support the venture, and whether or not these can viably be manipulated. It is advisable to work with those who are keen and supportive of the project, and who feel their personal backing will be of benefit. Investment of time, emotion, support, and effort is more likely to maintain interest and support.

'The second specific guideline refers to the social psychology of groups and the advantages of building teams of workers.'

The team should be self-sustaining and able to generate its own motivation and provide support for individual members. The group process will be facilitated if the members have approximately equal levels of skill and expertise and a shared ideology. Team cohesion should be maintained by not allowing team members to become isolated within the organization, especially by being expected to develop the service alone in a non-supportive or hostile environment. The team's functioning should also be facilitated by the organizational change manager, who should identify someone within the organization with which the team can work. This will create a liaison with the team and a supportive part of the organization's infrastructure.

'The organizational change manager should work with the healthy part of the system.'

'Healthy' refers to the parts of the organization that have potential to change. This means finding people who are keen, enthusiastic, and ambitious to produce a quality service, and avoiding those who are time-serving, resentful, or burnt out. It also applies to the organization: time should not be invested in areas of low morale and poor performance, since this will potentially stifle the development of the new service or project. Unhealthy parts of the organization rarely attract extra resources to rectify their problems or to encourage new developments. This in itself further encourages a resentful attitude on the part of the staff in these areas, who are unlikely to assist outsiders implementing a new service.

> *'It is advantagous to work with individuals and groups who have the authority or independence to make their own decisions.'*

This does not necessarily mean time should not be spent in groundwork with people who are not in senior positions, but that it is an uneconomic use of time and resources to spend a lot of effort in planning change with someone or some group who does not have the power to implement change. Determine where and how decisions are made, and if possible, plan changes with those who can implement them. Communicating plans for an intervention programme to service managers, and briefing them on the goals and benefits of such a programme may help to obtain their support and approval; it will at least avoid difficulties arising at a later date because they were not informed.

> *'It is recommended that appropriate levels of commitment and involvement be obtained from those in top management positions.'*

This strategy is to be strongly endorsed, and refers to the first and fourth points above. Backing from top management is essential, and commitment and involvement can frequently be obtained from someone who is ambitious and rising in the hierarchy. The greater involvement this person has with the service or project the better, since their commitment will vary with the amount of personal investment they have in the venture. Although day-to-day involvement from someone in such a senior management position may be low, their support is essential since they may have access to resource allocation or decision-making processes that team members and the organizational change manager do not have. Sometimes enlisting positive help or action is not possible, and benign indifference is the best that can be achieved, but even this condition is perfectly workable in many circumstances.

> *'Protect team members from stress and burnout.'*

The organizational change manager should deal with the negative reaction from the organization, which allows the team members to get on with the job of setting up and delivering the service. Similarly, avoidance of stress and burn-out can be achieved by: time off, such as conference and course attendance; variability of routine or some kind of work or task rotation; group and team support; and a team ethos that does not allow individuals to become isolated and alienated. The team should develop supportive mechanisms with which to protect individuals from extra stress.

SPECIALIST VS. GENERIC SERVICES

In setting up an intervention programme, a decision has to be made whether it will be a specialist service delivered by a specialist team, or a general service delivered widely by most personnel within the service. Although the idea of having the ability to deliver a family intervention as a core skill of all professions is attractive, at the present time it is probably premature.

The most workable system is one in which a small group of professionals concentrate on providing a specialist service. This allows a concentration of skills and ability, and a focus on helping families without the interference of other demands. Furthermore, a specialist service or team approach has a number of other advantages:

1. The danger of watering down the intervention skills to the lowest common denominator is avoided;
2. The possibility of producing real change is increased;
3. The concentration of skills avoids a 'patchy absorption' of skills found in training a large number of different professionals;
4. A small team with a specialist focus allows closer attainment of Georgiades and Phillimore's recommendations;
5. It increases the profile and perceived value of the programme;
6. It allows staff to develop specializations, and hence facilitates their career development.

From our experience, the best way to proceed is to set up a small specialist service of a core team of personnel who have at least part-time commitment to providing an intervention programme; have acquired specialist skills; are keen, enthusiastic, and supportive of one another; and who will contribute to the part of the service that most welcomes them.

PUBLIC RELATIONS

The necessity of good public relations cannot be sufficiently emphasized. In order to produce change so that an intervention programme can be initiated and maintained, it is necessary to know the structures and processes within the organization and how these function. This knowledge can then be used to positively promote the programme. A number of guidelines for achieving this aim follow.

Do the Appropriate Groundwork

Identify the people and healthy parts of the organization with which you can work. If possible, set the scene so there is a demand from within the organization for the programme, whereby others will be persuading you to set up the intervention, rather than you trying to persuade them. To do this requires the sowing of ideas widely within the organization, which can be carried out in a number of ways:

1. Inform and generate interest by talking to staff at all levels;
2. Invite outside experts to give lectures and seminars at your workplace; reactions will indicate who will and who will not be receptive of your ideas;
3. Foster the 'Why aren't we doing that here?' attitude;
4. Promote a top-down infusion of enthusiasm by outlining the benefits of family intervention programmes to senior members of staff and management;
5. Promote the benefits of the intervention in terms of interests to the person, for example, budget-holders may be interested in the economic savings, managers in the service evaluation aspects, and so on;
6. Identify all possible resources and allies to promote your programme, for example, consumer groups, relatives' support groups, and newly qualified professionals in training.

In summary, disseminate information and solicit assistance at all possible levels.

Identify Your Best Strategy
Be Ready to Put the Strategy into Action

Avoid promising too much or delaying too long before initiating the programme.

Maintain Good Public Relations

Inform those who have helped or taken an interest on your progress, keep them interested, and provide positive feedback. If you require active assistance from someone, keep in contact with them, for example, if you have got the co-operation of a ward or health centre staff, this will soon end if they never see or hear from you. Members of staff are much more likely to be co-operative if they know you and see you frequently.

Develop and foster good personal relationships at all levels. If you are cold and aloof; infrequently in contact, or only in contact when you want something; fail to follow up referrals; do not provide feedback or positive reinforcement to other staff in response to their help, then you will be much less likely to get and keep the co-operation of other staff.

Family intervention programmes require the assistance and co-operation of many staff who are not directly involved in the programme or part of the specialist team. Through the actions of other staff the intervention team will need to obtain referrals; be positively presented to the patient and their family; receive feedback and information from those in contact with the patient and family; obtain the co-operation of the responsible medical officer to get permission to implement the intervention; and to monitor and, if necessary, adjust medication.

To receive optimum co-operation and liaison, it is important to inform and update all such people on what you are doing. Ask each at what level they would like to be informed, foster those who show interest, discuss with them details of the cases they are also involved with, and solicit their opinion when appropriate.

In providing a new service such as a family intervention programme, whatever profession you come from, you will be crossing established professional boundaries, which will result in difficulties. This is virtually unavoidable, but the aim is to minimize the potential disruption to the programme. The suggestions above are possible ways of doing this. Some people in your organization will be antagonistic to the programme for one reason or another. Local knowledge of your workplace, and the attitudes of the various groups and individuals will help you to circumvent these problems. Some individuals may support your programme under some conditions but not under others, so try to provide the optimum conditions for your success.

If all these suggestions and discussion sound somewhat Machiavellian, that is because the strategies are goal-directed, and the desired outcome justifies the means of achievement. The aim is to set up and run a successful family intervention programme in order to bring the maximum benefit to the sufferers of schizophrenia and their families. This is likely to be achieved by bringing as many agendas as possible (including your own) in line with this aim.

OPERATIONAL STRATEGY

A broad strategy for setting up a family intervention programme follows, although this should be modified to take any local circumstances into account.

1. Familiarize yourself with the appropriate background information and specific knowledge required to carry out the intervention.
2. Identify possible team members and start to co-ordinate their activities.
3. Nominate the organizational change manager.
4. Obtain the support of your immediate superiors.
5. Obtain detailed information concerning the functioning of the organization.
6. Disseminate information about family interventions as widely and thoroughly as possible.
7. Formulate the structure and details of the intervention programme.
8. Inform and, if possible, obtain the support of senior management.
9. Identify with whom and in which part of the organization you intend to implement the programme.
10. Develop networks of close and distant collaborators, and foster personal relationships at all levels within that part of the organization.
11. Identify other resources or collaborators who may support or provide a positive influence on the programme.
12. Implement the programme at pilot level.
13. Maintain close links with all staff involved at a clinical level.
14. Inform widely within and outside the organization, of your initial aims and progress.
15. Evaluate your progress and take appropriate action to maintain your programme at optimal level.

Appendices

Relative Assessment Interview (RAI)

AIMS

This interview is designed for use in obtaining information from relatives about their experiences of coping with schizophrenic illness in a family member. The aims of the interview are:

1. To obtain information about the patient's psychiatric history, symptoms and behaviours, and social and role functioning.
2. To elicit the relative's response in terms of their behaviours, beliefs or thoughts, and subjective feelings, towards the patient and the illness; and the consequences of the illness related events to themselves and other members of the family. Here we are concerned to elicit positive and successful coping responses and resources of the family members, as well as areas of difficulty.

Unlike the Camberwell Family Interview, which is used to rate expressed emotion, this interview allows the interviewer to ask direct questions concerning the relatives' emotional reactions towards the patient. Topics which appear problematic should be probed extensively since this information may be used to identify areas of need. Specific examples of both the relative's and the patient's behaviour should be elicited.

STYLE OF INTERVIEW

The interviewer should attempt to become familiar with the interview schedule before carrying out the interview, since topics will come up out of order. An experienced interviewer can move around the schedule quite freely. The interviewer should use her or his judgement on the type and nature of the questions, but all areas should be covered. Questioning should begin with general questions, followed by specific questions to obtain more detailed information. The style of the interview should be relaxed and conversational and not time limited, with the interviewer giving empathic feedback that they are listening and understanding what the relative has to say.

Usually, relatives welcome the opportunity to speak at length about their experiences. The interviewer should adopt an approach that fosters a collaborative endeavour, whereby the interviewer and respondent work together to obtain the information necessary to identify problems and begin to work on resolving difficulties.

Remember that the interview schedule is a guide to the interview, and not a checklist.

Background Information

Composition of Household

Who lives in the household? If the patient does not live with the respondent, then where and with whom does he/she live?

Elicit details about those who live with or who have contact with the patient, such as their age, sex, relationship to the patient, current education or employment status, including such details for the respondent and the patient, if they are not already available.

Contact Time

How does the patient usually spend his/her day? How much contact does the relative have with the patient on a typical day?

Try to elicit how many hours each day the patient and the relative are in direct contact with each other (i.e. in the same room) and the nature of this contact, for example, what do they do together, do they talk or interact in some other way, or are they performing separate activities? Enquire whether the patterns differ throughout the week, such as between weekdays and weekends. Where possible, follow up any leads about how the respondent feels about the frequency and nature of their interactions with the patient, for example, how they get along when together.

Similarly, ask about who else the patient sees, how frequently, and for how long. It can be helpful to ask direct questions about specific periods during the days, such as, meal times, evenings, etc., and how various household members spend their time or come together.

Psychiatric History (A)

Complete Psychiatric History

Obtain a brief chronological account of the whole history of psychiatric illness. Include approximate dates and duration of episodes. Useful questions include:

When did the patient's trouble first begin?
When did the respondent first notice something different about him/her?
When did the respondent first realize there was something wrong?
When was the patient last his/her normal self?
Was there a sudden or gradual deterioration?
How long has the patient's problem been going on?
How did the respondent and others react? When the problems began?
What was the patient's reaction to his/her problem and its development?
(For each symptom or problem spontaneously mentioned by the relative, ask about onset, severity, context, reactions, how the relative felt, etc.)

Current Episode (for Relapse or Acutely Ill Patients) or Recent Illness History

When the patient has had a recent relapse, obtain similar information as identified above about the current episode – its beginning and development. If no current episode, ask about patient's condition over the last three months. For relapse patients, useful questions include:

Did the patient go into hospital this last time? Or see the doctor or other professional?
When did the patient begin to get worse?
What did he/she do?
What happened?
How did the patient feel about coming to the hospital? Or seeing the doctor?
How did he/she behave?

Ask the respondent to describe the events around the admission and how the patient and others, including the respondent, reacted to this. Ask directly about the relative's thoughts feelings and behaviours in response to symptoms and problems. What were the effects and consequences of any coping strategies? Look for examples of attempts to 'control' the patient's behaviour and elicit details.

For Patients Who Have Not Recently Relapsed
Could you tell me how the patient has been getting along in the past three months?
Generally speaking, do you think they have shown improvement, or got worse, or stayed about the same?

Pinpoint areas of improvement or deterioration, that is, identify specific behavioural examples, and elicit the relative's thoughts feelings and behaviours in response to the patient's improved or deteriorated behaviour.

Psychiatric Symptoms (A) (Have the Symptoms Occurred in the Last Three Months?)

Patient Irritability
Enquire about any examples of the patient being irritable, snappy, losing their temper, and so on. ('Are there any times when ---- gets irritable or snappy?')
What would happen: would they shout? Swear? Get impatient? Quarrel? Argue?

Ask how frequently this would occur, and elicit details by asking the respondent to describe one or two specific examples. What precipitated this sort of reaction in the patient? When did it happen? Who was there? How did they react? How similar/dissimilar are the situations described by the relative to other situations when the patient is irritable? Has the patient got more irritable/less irritable in the past three months?

When the patient behaves like this how do family members behave/feel? How does the respondent behave/feel?

If the respondent reports no irritability in the patient in the last three months, ask whether the patient ever gets cross or impatient, or, if so, why? Can the respondent remember the last time the patient lost their temper or became irritable?

Tension in the Household and Irritability of Other Family Members

If the relative has suggested that arguments and quarrels do occur, elicit whether they result in an atmosphere of tension in the household. If so, how is this apparent? Does it affect people visiting the house? Or cause anyone to avoid the house or stay away? Who is involved and what do they do in the situation?

Probe for all family members to find out if there are any arguments or disputes because of the patient, or concerning other matters. In most families there are disagreements from time to time. How do the rest of the family get along together? Are there any times when family members argue or get on at one another? Which family members? What are the arguments about? What about the respondent? Are they involved in the disagreements? How do they feel/behave?

Nagging, Grumbling, and Irritability of Other Family Members

Do you ever get irritable or snappy with the patient? Or nag (moan, grumble) at them? For what reasons? What sorts of things are complained about? What about other members of the family (specify by name)? (If there is some irritability towards the patient, ask about the context, frequency, outcomes, etc.) Ask also about any irritability, nagging or moaning between other family members about the patient.

Query whether there has been any change in irritability or nagging over the past three months, and if so, for what reason.

Psychiatric History (B)

Instructions

This section of questioning is important for establishing the patient's symptom profile; for understanding which areas of the patient's functioning are problematic for the relative or family members; for learning about the relative's understanding about the illness and the symptoms as well as how they cope with difficulties; and what consequences the problems have had on the individual relative and the family as a whole.

1. Ask all specified questions unless full information on the relevant behaviour collected in Section A.
2. Use this section to obtain a picture of pattern of severity of illness during primary period – if not done in Section A.

In order to get a detailed behavioural description for each symptom, some useful general probes are:

Onset	When did this first begin?
	Has it occurred during the last three months?
Severity	How did this show itself? (obtain example)
	At worst, what was this behaviour/ideas/like
Frequency	How often did . . . happen?
	Did it happen all the time? Every day?
	Once a week? Etc.
Social Context	Where did it happen? Who was there? What time of day?
Reactions	How did you react?
	What effect did this have on you/how did you feel about it? (Similarly for the reactions of others).
Tension	Does/did it make you feel on edge?
	Is/was there an atmosphere in the home?
Legitimacy	Do you have any ideas why he/she behaves like that/ does that?
	Is this behaviour different from his/her normal self, how he/she used to be before the illness?
	Do you think he/she could do/have done any more to control it?

Coping	How did you deal with . . . ?
	How effective was this?
	Did you find any way of preventing it? Or making the situation better?

Introduce topic

'I'd like to ask some questions about the way [the patient] may have been affected by this trouble. I'll go through some of the symptoms or difficulties that we sometimes see in people who have [the patient's] kind of problem. Of course, some won't apply, but I would like to run through all of these and perhaps you'd tell me whether or not he/she has been like this, particularly in the last three months.'

Bodily functions

Sleep	Has the patient had any difficulties with his/her sleep recently? Such as, any difficulty in getting off? Nightmares? Waking up very early?
Appetite	Ask whether the patient has had any difficulties/changes with his/her appetite.

Physical Complaints

Has he/she complained of any physical problems, such as, headaches, dizziness, any other aches or pains?

Activity

Underactivity	Has the patient been inactive or lacking in energy for example, doing less, sitting around, not helping out around the house? Etc. How different is this from the patient's past levels of activity?
Slowness	Has he/she seemed particularly slow in doing everyday things, for example, dressing (shaving), making beds, washing up, etc.
Overactivity	Query whether there have been times when the patient has been unusually active, for example, has he/she had times of being unusually cheerful? Or of being excited or agitated? Or of being noisy or shouting a lot?

	Talkative? Or swearing? Or of being rude? Or of being restless – such as pacing about?
Violence	Have there been episodes of violence? What happened and to whom? Was anyone hit or hurt? Did you feel frightened? How did you cope with the situation?
	Do you feel threatened at present or worry that he/she could be violent again in the future?
Destructive behaviour	Have there ever been incidents when property or objects have been broken?
Withdrawal	Has the patient had periods of being withdrawn or avoiding people? Have they been especially quiet at home? Or avoided going out? Or avoided seeing people when they come to the house?
Fears/Anxiety	Has the patient had periods of being afraid or anxious? Ask how the respondent knew that this was so? Did the patient stop doing things or change in anyway because of their fears? How did others react to the patient when they were like this?
Worry	Has the patient been worrying about anything recently? If so, what? How does the respondent know the patient was worrying? Has the patient talked about his/her concerns? What happened? How did the respondent deal with this?
Overt Misery	Ask whether the patient has been depressed? Miserable? Tearful? Said that life is not worth living? Blamed him/herself? Tried to harm him/herself? How did the patient complain about feeling this way? How did the relative respond and how did they feel when the patient told them? Have you been worried that the patient may harm him/herself or attempt to end their life?
Obsessions	Ask whether the patient has been unusually fussy or finicky about anything?, like being very concerned about germs or cleanliness? Or has had routines of doing things only in a certain way, even though it seems silly? Or doing things over and over again? – like washing his/her hands, or keep checking that the door is locked?

Personal Care   Does the patient look after her/himself?
                           Keep himself clean and tidy? Wash and
                           dress appropriately, etc.? Has this changed?
                           Compared to others, e.g. siblings?

Delusions/Hallucinations Ask whether the patient has expressed any
                           strange ideas, and if so what about? Has he/
                           she thought people were against him/her?
                           Has he/she had strange ideas about anyone
                           in the family? Said that anything strange
                           or odd was going on? Accused people of
                           anything? Or said that there was anything
                           unusual affecting him/her? Or that there
                           was anything strange about the TV, food and
                           drink, the neighbours, etc.?
                           Has he/she appeared to be acting in a strange
                           way? Talking or laughing to himself/herself?
                           Adopting strange mannerisms or postures?
                           How has this affected him/her?
                           What have you said to her/him about this?
                           What happened when you said/did this?
                           Has anyone else at home said/done anything?

Bizarre Behaviour   Ask whether the patient has done any-
                           thing else that seemed strange or bizarre or
                           unusual for him/her?
                             Has her/his behaviour seemed different
                           in anyway? Such as wandering off from
                           home? Has he/she been drinking a lot? . . . or
                           gambling a lot?

Household Tasks

Ask about the various household tasks such as shopping, cleaning,
cooking, gardening, repairs, etc. Who does them? Has this situation
changed recently or in association with any other change in the patient's
behaviour? Is the respondent satisfied with the situation? If not, has
he/she tried to do anything about it and with what result?

Who does the various jobs around the house? (Specify who does what)
Does the patient help out with . . . ?
What sort of things does the patient do?
Has the way he/she has done the task changed since his/her troubles
    began? If so, how?
Does he/she do it as well as before?
When did the change occur?
What seemed to be the reason for this?

Do you do them together?
Are you satisfied with the way things are done at home?
Why not?
Does this ever lead to disagreements?

Money Matters

Find out how well the patient handles money and whether there have been any changes. What are the problems? Who handles the household finances? Does the patient pay towards his/her keep? Is the respondent satisfied with this arrangement? If not probe further. What would the respondent like to happen?

Ask about any changes in the household's finances since the patient became ill. Has her/his illness caused any financial burden or hardship? Has the relative had to make any sacrifices because of the patient? For example, if the relative has given up work to be with the patient have there been financial difficulties because of this? How does the relative feel about this? How have the difficulties been manifest, e.g. not paying the rent/bills, getting into debt, use of credit card, cutting down on spending, etc.?

Since most people are quite sensitive about talking about their personal finances these questions should be asked with care and sensitivity.

Interests and Activities of the Relative

Introduction of questioning: 'I'd like to ask you a few questions about how you spend your time, what your interests are and so on, and any ways in which these things have changed since [the patient] has been ill.'

Employment: if employed, nature of the work, and number of hours employed.

Leisure: how does the relative spend their leisure time/what are their interests/hobbies.

Social supports outside the immediate family: outside of the household, are there any friends/relatives/people who the respondent sees regularly? Is the respondent able to talk to them freely about any problems that come up at home? Do they find this helpful?

In parental household: how much time do you and your husband/wife spend together? What sorts of things do you do/enjoy doing together? Do you find it helpful to talk problems over with your husband/wife? If yes, how does it help? If no, why not, and is there anyone else you find it helpful to talk to?

Changes in Interests, Occupations and Social Activities

Have you found that there have been changes in the way you spend your
time since (the patient's) problems first began?
For example with work? with activities? with seeing friends? with the
time you spend with your husband/wife?
Why have the changes taken place?
What does the relative feel about them?

Relationship with Patient

Obtain information about the relative's relationship with the patient and
any changes due to the illness.

Ask how the relative and patient get on?
Do you find him/her a friendly person?
Is he/she easy to get on with?
Can you get close to him/her?
In what ways would you like him/her to be different?
In what ways does he/she get on your nerves?
Ask whether the relative ever talks to the patient about these complaints
Ask whether the relative has avoided or kept out of the patient's way?
Why?
Has the respondent felt any differently towards the patient?
Has the amount of affection for the patient changed? In what way?

Elicit any change in the relationship on the part of the patient.

Has he/she behaved any differently towards you since this trouble
started?
Has the amount of affection he/she has shown to you changed? or the
amount of interest he/she has shown in you?
In general how would you say you got on together?
Can you tell when he or she is upset or happy?
Do you think he/she can tell when you are upset or happy?

Elicit any large changes in the relative's behaviour or feelings since the
illness began.

What difference has her/his illness made to you and the family?
From your point of view, what is the most disturbing aspect of her/his
troubles?

Final Question

Is there anything else I have not covered or you would like to tell me?
Thank the relative for their co-operation.

Family Questionnaire (FQ)

We are interested in finding out what problems, if any, you experience with your relative at home. We would also like to find out how much stress these problems cause you and how well you feel able to cope with the difficulties. We hope this information will be of use in helping relatives to overcome such problems.

Please read each statement which describes a behaviour which may have occurred with your relative. If it has not occurred simply circle the '1' in the first column to indicate that this behaviour never happens. There is no need to mark the other two columns in this case.

However, if the behaviour does occur, please indicate how often it does so by circling one of the numbers. For example, if your relative 'becomes irritable and easily upset' several times each week, then circle the 4 to show that this happens frequently. In much the same way, please indicate in the next two columns how much this behaviour bothers you, and how well or badly you feel able to cope with it at home.

How often does this happen?	How much does this bother you?	How well do you feel able to control and cope with this behaviour?
1 = never 2 = rarely 3 = sometimes 4 = frequently 5 = always	1 = not at all 2 = a little 3 = moderately 4 = quite a lot 5 = considerably	1 = not at all 2 = fairly badly 3 = adequately 4 = reasonably well 5 = as well as possible

	How often does this happen?	How much does this bother you?	How well do you feel able to control and cope with this behaviour?
Becomes restless e.g. pacing about, not sitting through meals.	1 2 3 4 5	1 2 3 4 5	1 2 3 4 5
Complains of headaches or other pains.	1 2 3 4 5	1 2 3 4 5	1 2 3 4 5
Is unpredictable or impulsive.	1 2 3 4 5	1 2 3 4 5	1 2 3 4 5
Hits or hurts people.	1 2 3 4 5	1 2 3 4 5	1 2 3 4 5
Gets noisy or shouts a lot.	1 2 3 4 5	1 2 3 4 5	1 2 3 4 5
Is unusually fussy or finicky about things.	1 2 3 4 5	1 2 3 4 5	1 2 3 4 5
Gets bored very easily or has difficulty occupying himself/herself.	1 2 3 4 5	1 2 3 4 5	1 2 3 4 5
Gets jealous of other members of the family or friends.	1 2 3 4 5	1 2 3 4 5	1 2 3 4 5
Lacks interest in friends and relatives.	1 2 3 4 5	1 2 3 4 5	1 2 3 4 5
Is odd in appearance, manner or movement.	1 2 3 4 5	1 2 3 4 5	1 2 3 4 5
Avoids meeting people.	1 2 3 4 5	1 2 3 4 5	1 2 3 4 5
Gets destructive or knocks things about in the house.	1 2 3 4 5	1 2 3 4 5	1 2 3 4 5
Talks to himself/herself or imaginary companions.	1 2 3 4 5	1 2 3 4 5	1 2 3 4 5
Wakes/gets up unusually early in the morning.	1 2 3 4 5	1 2 3 4 5	1 2 3 4 5
Grumbles a lot.	1 2 3 4 5	1 2 3 4 5	1 2 3 4 5
Sits or lies around not doing much.	1 2 3 4 5	1 2 3 4 5	1 2 3 4 5
Thinks people are against him/her.	1 2 3 4 5	1 2 3 4 5	1 2 3 4 5
Lacks concentration and attention.	1 2 3 4 5	1 2 3 4 5	1 2 3 4 5
Slow at doing things.	1 2 3 4 5	1 2 3 4 5	1 2 3 4 5
Stays out very late at night.	1 2 3 4 5	1 2 3 4 5	1 2 3 4 5
Becomes irritable and easily upset.	1 2 3 4 5	1 2 3 4 5	1 2 3 4 5
Is unclean and untidy.	1 2 3 4 5	1 2 3 4 5	1 2 3 4 5
Spends long periods alone.	1 2 3 4 5	1 2 3 4 5	1 2 3 4 5
Has marked difficulties with memory, such as not being able to find his/her way home, difficulty remembering people's houses.	1 2 3 4 5	1 2 3 4 5	1 2 3 4 5
Expresses odd ideas.	1 2 3 4 5	1 2 3 4 5	1 2 3 4 5
Has unusual fears.	1 2 3 4 5	1 2 3 4 5	1 2 3 4 5

Continued

Is unusually cheerful or excited.	1 2 3 4 5	1 2 3 4 5	1 2 3 4 5
Talks or laughs to himself/herself.	1 2 3 4 5	1 2 3 4 5	1 2 3 4 5
Says nothing when spoken to.	1 2 3 4 5	1 2 3 4 5	1 2 3 4 5
Fritters money away.	1 2 3 4 5	1 2 3 4 5	1 2 3 4 5
Abuses drugs.	1 2 3 4 5	1 2 3 4 5	1 2 3 4 5
Drinks excessively.	1 2 3 4 5	1 2 3 4 5	1 2 3 4 5
Has difficulty in getting to sleep	1 2 3 4 5	1 2 3 4 5	1 2 3 4 5
Has unusual habits or routines, e.g. in dressing, or hoarding strange things.	1 2 3 4 5	1 2 3 4 5	1 2 3 4 5
Has poor appetite/does not want to eat.	1 2 3 4 5	1 2 3 4 5	1 2 3 4 5
Has routines of doing things only in a certain way.	1 2 3 4 5	1 2 3 4 5	1 2 3 4 5
Keeps to himself/herself a lot.	1 2 3 4 5	1 2 3 4 5	1 2 3 4 5
Accuses or threatens people.	1 2 3 4 5	1 2 3 4 5	1 2 3 4 5
Has periods of panic or anxiety.	1 2 3 4 5	1 2 3 4 5	1 2 3 4 5
Acts in a bizarre way.	1 2 3 4 5	1 2 3 4 5	1 2 3 4 5
Has rows or quarrels.	1 2 3 4 5	1 2 3 4 5	1 2 3 4 5
Worries a lot about things.	1 2 3 4 5	1 2 3 4 5	1 2 3 4 5
Swears or is rude to people.	1 2 3 4 5	1 2 3 4 5	1 2 3 4 5
Gets miserable and depressed.	1 2 3 4 5	1 2 3 4 5	1 2 3 4 5
Pays insufficient towards keep.	1 2 3 4 5	1 2 3 4 5	1 2 3 4 5
Talks nonsense when spoken to.	1 2 3 4 5	1 2 3 4 5	1 2 3 4 5
Mixes with undesirable company.	1 2 3 4 5	1 2 3 4 5	1 2 3 4 5
Refuses to take medication (tablets or injections).	1 2 3 4 5	1 2 3 4 5	1 2 3 4 5
Any other problems (please specify).			

Thank you very much for your help

Social Functioning Scale (SFS)*

*(Printed with the kind permission of Dr Max Birchwood)

Name_____ Date_____

SUMMARY OF SCORES

Sub-Section	Transformed Scores
Social Withdrawal	_____
Interpersonal Functioning	_____
Prosocial Activities	_____
Recreation	_____
Level of Independence Competence	_____
Performance	_____
Employment	_____
Total Score (Mean)	_____

SECTION ONE: WITHDRAWAL

Part One

1. What time does (s)he get up each day?

   Average weekday [ ]

   Average weekend (if different) [ ]

   3: <9 am
   2: 9 am to 11 am
   1: 11 am to 1 pm
   0: >1 pm

2. How many hours of the waking day does (s)he spend alone?
   (e.g. on own in room, walking out alone, listening to radio or watching TV alone, etc.)?
   Count the number of hours in an average day spent alone and tick (√) one of the following.

   Hours spent alone

   (√)

0–3	Very little time spent alone.	[ ]	3
3–6	Some of the time.	[ ]	2
6–9	Quite a lot of the time.	[ ]	1
9–12	A great deal of time.	[ ]	0
12–	Practically all the time.	[ ]	

3. How often will (s)he start a conversation at home?

       0   1   2   3

   Almost never / rarely / sometimes / often   (underline)

4. How often will (s)he leave the house (for any reason)?

       0   1   2   3

   Almost never / rarely / sometimes / often   (underline)

5. How does (s)he react to the presence of strangers?

       0   1   2   3

   Avoids them / feels nervous / accepts them / likes them   (underline)

INTERPERSONAL FUNCTIONING

Part Two

1. How many friends does (s)he have at the moment? (persons whom (s)he will see regularly, do activities with, etc.)

   Number of friends

2. Has (s)he someone (s)he finds it easy to discuss feelings and difficulties with?

   3   0
   YES/NO

3. How often has (s)he confided in them?

   0   1   2   3
   Almost never / rarely / sometimes / often

4. Do other people discuss their problems with him/her?

   0   1   2   3
   Almost never / rarely / sometimes / often

5. Does (s)he have a boy/girl-friend? (If not married)

   (If married = 3)

   3   0
   YES/NO

6. Has (s)he had any arguments with friends, relatives or neighbours recently?

   3   2   1   0
   None / 1 or 2 minor / continued minor or 1 major/ many major

7. How often are you able to carry out a sensible or rational conversation with him/her

   0   1   2   3
   Almost never / rarely / sometimes / often

8. How easy or difficult does (s)he find it talking to people at the moment?

   3   2   2   0   0
   Very easy / quite easy / average / quite difficult / very difficult

9. Does (s)he feel uneasy with groups of people?

   3   2   1   0
   Almost never / rarely / sometimes / often

10. Does (s)he out of preference spend time on his/her own?

    0   1   2   3
    Often / somtimes / rarely / almost never

PRO-SOCIAL ACTIVITIES

Part Three

Put a tick (√) in the appropriate column to show how often (s)he has
participated in any of the following activities *over the past three months*.

	0 Never	1 Rarely	2 Sometimes	3 Often
Cinema				
Theatre/concert, etc.				
Watching an indoor sport .... (e.g. squash, table-tennis)				
Watching an outdoor sport .... (e.g. football, rugby)				
Art gallery/Museum.				
Exhibition				
Visiting places of interest				
Meeting, talk, etc.				
Evening class.				

Continued

	0 Never	1 Rarely	1 Sometimes	3 Often
Visiting relatives in their homes				
Being visited by relative.				
Visiting friends (including boy/girlfriend)				
Being visited by friends (including boy/girlfriend)				
Parties				
Formal occasions				
Disco, etc.				
Night club/social club				
Playing an outdoor sport				
Club/society....................................				
Pub..				
Eating out				
Church activity................................				

Any other activity?	Rarely	Sometimes	Often
_____			
_____			
_____			

SECTION TWO: RECREATION ACTIVITIES

Please place a tick in the appropriate column to indicate how often (s)he has done any of the following activities *over the past 3 months.*

	0	1	2	3
	Never	Rarely	Sometimes	Often
Playing musical instruments				
Sewing, knitting				
Gardening				
Reading things				
Watching television				
Listening to records or radio				
Cooking				
DIY activities				
Fixing things (car, bike, household, etc.)				
Walking/rambling				
Driving/cycling (as a recreation)				
Swimming				
Hobby (e.g. collecting things)				
Shopping				
Artistic activity (painting, crafts, etc.)				

Any other recreation or pastime?

	Rarely 1	Sometimes 2	Often 3
_____			
_____			
_____			

SECTION THREE: INDEPENDENCE (C)

Please place a tick against each item to show how able (s)he is at doing or using the following:

	3 *Adequately* (no help)	2 *Needs help* (or prompting)	1 *Unable* (or without lots of help)	0 *Not known*
Public transport				
Handling money correctly				
Budgetting				
Cooking for self				
Weekly shopping				
How to look for a job				
Washing own clothes				
Personal hygiene				
Washing, tidying, etc.				
Purchasing from shops				
Leaving the house alone				
Choosing and buying own clothes				
Taking care of personal appearance				

Independence (P)

Please place a tick against each item to show how often (s)he has done the following *over the past three months*.

	0 Never	1 Rarely	2 Sometimes	3 Often
Buying items from shops alone (without help)				
Washing pots, tidying up, etc.				
Regular washing, bathing, etc.				
Washing own clothes				
Looking for a job (if unemployed)				
Doing the food shopping				
Prepare and cook a meal				
Leaving the house alone				
Using buses, trains, etc.				
Using money				
Budgetting				
Choosing and buying clothes for self				
Takes care of personal appearance				

SECTION FOUR: EMPLOYMENT

1. Is (s)he in regular employment (including industrial therapy, rehabilitation or re-training courses)?

    Yes / No   (underline)

    If yes: What sort of job?   _____

    _____

    How many hours does (s)he work each week?   _____

    How long has (s)he had this job?   _____

    If no :   When was (s)he last in employment?   _____

    What sort of job was it?   _____

    _____

    How many hours per week?   _____

2. If not employed:
    Is (s)he registered disabled?   Yes / No   (underline)

    Does (s)he attend hospital as a day-patient?
    Yes / No   (underline)

    Do you think (s)he is capable of some sort of employment?
    Definitely yes / would have difficulty / definitely no

    How often does (s)he make attempts to find a job (e.g. go to Job Centre, look in newspaper, etc.)?
    Almost never / rarely / sometimes / often

3. If not employed:
    How does (s)he usually occupy his/her day?

    Morning: _____

    Afternoon: _____

    Evening: _____

SOCIAL ADJUSTMENT SCALES
SCALED SCORE EQUIVALENT OF RAW SCORES
MEAN:100 S.D.:15
SCALED SCORES

RAW SCORES

SCALE SCORE	With-drawal	Inter-action	Pro-social	Rec-reation	Independ-ence (p)	Independ-ence (c)	Occupa-tional
0	57.5	55	65.0	57.0			81.5
1	65.0	78	76.0	63.0	53.0		89.5
2	70.5	86	79.0	66.0	56.5		95.0
3	75.5	91	83.0	69.0	60.0		97.5
4	80.0	96	86.0	72.0	63.5		103.0
5	84.0	100	88.5	74.5	67.5		107.0
6	87.5	105	91.0	77.0	70.0		109.5
7	90.5	111	93.5	80.0	71.5		112.5
8	93.5	124	95.0	81.5	73.5		114.0
9	96.5	145	96.5	84.0	75.0		116.0
10	100.0		98.0	86.5	76.5	55.0	122.5
11	104.5		100.0	89.0	78.0	58.0	
12	110.0		101.5	91.0	79.0	61.0	
13	116.5		103.0	93.5	80.0	64.0	
14	124.5		105.0	96.0	81.5	66.5	
15	133.0		107.0	98.0	83.0	69.0	
16			108.5	101.0	84.5	72.5	
17			110.0	103.0	85.5	75.0	
18			111.5	105.5	87.5	76.5	
19			112.5	108.5	89.0	78.0	
20			114.5	110.5	90.5	79.5	
21			116.0	113.0	92.0	81.5	
22			117.5	116.5	94.0	83.0	
23			119.0	119.0	97.0	84.5	
24			121.0	121.5	100.5	86.5	
25			123.0	124.5	103.5	88.5	
26			124.0	126.5	105.5	90.5	
27			125.0	129.0	106.5	91.5	
28			126.0	131.0	107.0	93.0	
29			127.0	133.0	108.0	94.5	
30			128.0	135.0	109.0	95.5	
31			129.0	137.0	110.0	96.5	
32			129.5	139.0	112.5	97.5	
33			130.0	140.0	114.5	100.5	
34			130.5	142.0	116.5	103.5	
35			131.0	144.0	118.5	107.0	
36			131.5	145.0	121.5	110.0	
37			132.0		124.0	114.0	
38			132.5		127.0	117.5	
39			133.0		131.0	125.0	
40			133.5				
41			134.0				
42			135.0				
43			136.0				
44			137.0				
45			138.0				
46			139.0				
47			141.0				
48			142.0				
49			143.0				
50			145.0				

Personal Functioning Scale (PFS)

Ask about general level of functioning on each category over the last month. Rating is made from the informant's account. Try to get a general or average rating over the month and not specific accounts. Similarly try to rate generally over the whole area.

GENERAL COMMENTS

The aim of the rating is to get a quick global rating from the relative's or informant's perception of the patient. The rating is therefore subjective, probes can be added to verify that the informant understands what is required. The perception is a generalized one over the last month so if the informant gives excessive detail attempt to elicit an average rating, e.g. say *'yes, but generally over the last month how has X been?'*

To rate an extreme score, e.g., very bad or very good the informant should emphasize the extreme spontaneously.

The ratings are of four different areas:

1. General household activities
2. General sociability and manner
3. Activities outside the family
4. Overall behaviour

Each is rated on three dimensions:

1. *Level* – quantity of time spent on each or frequency of occurrence
2. *Change* – the difference between the last month and the month previous on level
3. The relative's *satisfaction* with the displayed level

Ratings should be made reasonably quickly without excessive concentration on detail.

1. Household Activities

Rate level of participation, i.e., quantity or frequency in the following areas:

a) Participation in household tasks or routines as would be appropriate for that person's role and expectations;
b) Participation in family activities, e.g., joint activities usually expected of a family, e.g., meals together, recreation, watching T.V.
c) Participation in decision processes, i.e., independence skills, acts as an autonomous unit within the family.

Probe questions:

Level: 'How much has X been helping out in household routines and jobs over the last month? Has X been joining in family activities such as meals? What else does X do?'

Rating

1. very bad:	no or only residual participation
2. poor:	little, not much or spasmodic
3. moderate:	occasional, reasonable or very variable
4. good:	quite frequent
5. very good:	participates nearly all the time or as required

Change

'Has this changed from the previous month? How?'

Rating:
1. greatly deteriorated
2. some deterioration
3. no change
4. some improvement
5. greatly improved

Satisfaction: 'Over the last month how satisfied have you been with this?'

Rating:

1. very bad:	very unsatisfied
2. poor:	unsatisfied
3. moderate:	reasonable
4. good:	satisfied
5. very good:	very satisfied

2. General Attitude

Type of participation, i.e., quality of social interaction in the house, e.g.:

a) sociable behaviour within normal limits, e.g., initiates greetings and conversations, responds to similar;

b) does not act in an aggressive or beligerent manner without reason, or out of context or in an excessive manner to mild provocation;
c) displays normal non-verbal behaviour, e.g., gestures, expressions, smiling, etc;
d) acts in a manner appropriate to social stimuli in both nature and intensity.

Probe questions:

Level: 'What has X's general manner and attitude been like over the last month? For example, has X been generally sociable and acting in a reasonable way?'

Rating
(As before)

Change

'Has this been a change from the previous month? How?'

Rating
(As before)

Satisfaction

'How satisfied have you been with this over the last month?'

Rating
(As before)

3. Social Activities

Level of participation in activities outside the family circle (quantity). Includes activities with others, e.g., friends, solitary activities with the aim of meeting others, e.g., singles clubs, etc., solitary activities without the main aim of meeting others but where this might happen due to a shared interest, e.g., fishing, sports, etc., include hetrosexual activities if with a boy or girlfriend, but not spouse or co-habitee or close relative.

Probe question:

Level: 'Generally over the last month, how well has X been at going out, meeting friends and socialising. Does X have interests or hobbies that he spends time doing away from home. Has X tried to find friends or get out?'

Rating
(As before)

Change

'Has this been a change from the previous month? In what way?'

Rating
(As before)

Satisfaction

'How satisfied (happy) have you been with this over the last month?'

Rating
(As before)

4. Overall Behaviour

All of patients behaviour. Includes global and general impression.

Probe question:

Level: 'Overall over the past months how do you think X has behaved? Generally, over the past month, how do you think X has been getting on?'

Rating
(As before)

Change
'Has this been a change from the previous month? In what way?'

Rating
(As before)

Satisfaction

'Generally how happy (satisfied) have you been with this over the last month?'

Rating
(As before)

SCORING SHEET

Household Activities

Level
1   Very Bad
2   Poor
3   Moderate
4   Good
5   Very Good

Change
1   Much Worse
2   Worse
3   No Change
4   Better
5   Much Better

Satisfaction
1   Very Bad
2   Poor
3   Moderate
4   Good
5   Very Good

General Attitude

Level
1   Very Bad
2   Poor
3   Moderate
4   Good
5   Very Good

Change
1   Much Worse
2   Worse
3   No Change
4   Better
5   Much Better

Satisfaction
1   Very Bad
2   Poor
3   Moderate
4   Good
5   Very Good

Social Activities (Outside of Family)

Level
1   Much Worse
2   Worse
3   No Change
4   Better
5   Much Better

Change
1   Much Worse
2   Worse
3   No Change
4   Better
5   Much Better

Satisfaction
1   Very Bad
2   Poor
3   Moderate
4   Good
5   Very Good

Overall Behaviour

Level
1   Very Bad
2   Poor
3   Moderate
4   Good
5   Very Good

Change
1   Much Worse
2   Worse
3   No Change
4   Better
5   Much Better

Satisfaction
1   Very Bad
2   Poor
3   Moderate
4   Good
5   Very Good

Knowledge About Schizophrenia Interview (KASI)

INTRODUCTION

I'd like to ask you some questions about . . .'s admission to hospital, what you know about the reasons for it; what . . . was treated for; what the treatment was and so on.

This is to help us give you and other relatives any information about your relative's condition that you might need. We just want to find out what you think or know already.

SECTION 1: DIAGNOSIS

1:1 What have you been told by the doctors/nurses or other people about the kind of problem that . . . was treated for?

(Question if necessary to identify source) . . . .

. . . .

. . . .

. . . . Source: . . . .

1:2 (If a diagnosis is not given): Do you know the name of the problem/diagnosis?

. . . .

1:3 (If answers to 1:1, and 1:2 are inadequate): What kind of problem do you think . . . was treated for?

. . . .

. . . .

1:4 (If gives some diagnosis): What do you understand by (insert name of problem given). Do you think it is:

	YES	NO	DON'T KNOW
(a) Having a minor nervous condition, or having been 'overdoing it' lately?	☐	☐	☐
(b) A severe mental illness which can affect all aspects of a person's life?	☐	☐	☐
(c) Other (specify . . . .).	☐	☐	☐

SECTION 2: SYMPTOMATOLOGY

2:1 You have mentioned that...'s problems affected her/him by: (*List 'symptoms' that the relative has mentioned in the RAI or other interviews) Do you think that this is...'s natural self, or do you think its part of '(insert name of problem given)'?

	Natural Self	Illness	Don't Know
(a)	☐	☐	☐
(b)	☐	☐	☐
(c)	☐	☐	☐
(d)	☐	☐	☐
(e)	☐	☐	☐

2:2 Do you know of any other ways in which she/he was affected e.g. strange ideas or difficulties with her/his thinking?

....
....

2:3 Do you think ... could help or control '.............................'
repeat 'symptoms' listed in 2:1 and elicited in 2:2?

	YES	NO	DON'T KNOW
(a)	☐	☐	☐
(b)	☐	☐	☐
(c)	☐	☐	☐
(d)	☐	☐	☐
(e)	☐	☐	☐
(f)	☐	☐	☐
(g)	☐	☐	☐
(h)	☐	☐	☐

2:4 Do you know the most common and important symptoms (difficulties) of people who have '(insert whatever relative calls person's illness)'?

....
....

*See Barrowclough et al., 1987.

2:5 Do you think the most common and important symptoms are:

	YES	NO	DON'T KNOW
(a) Hallucinations – hearing, seeing or smelling things which others can't hear, see or smell.	☐	☐	☐
(b) delusions – totally false beliefs others don't share.	☐	☐	☐
(c) disturbances of thinking such as thoughts being put into your head or broadcast to other people.	☐	☐	☐

SECTION 3: AETIOLOGY

3:1 What do you think is the cause of . . .'s '(insert whatever relative calls person's illness)'?

....

....

....

....

3:2 Do you think any of the following might have caused it?

	YES	NO	DON'T KNOW
(a) A biological illness affecting the way the brain works?	☐	☐	☐
(b) The way someone is brought up? (e.g. having an unhappy childhood)	☐	☐	☐
(c) It is inherited (runs in families)?	☐	☐	☐
(d) (add causes mentioned by relative)	☐	☐	☐

....

3:3 Of all things just mentioned; what do you think is the main cause?

....

....

3:4 *Ask only if relative gives an 'incorrect' answer to any of previous questions in this section:*
You said that you think . . . may cause 'insert relatives name for condition.' Is there anything you might do to help remedy this/sort this out?

....

....

SECTION 4: MEDICATION

4:1 Has the doctor or psychiatrist prescribed any tablets or injections for . . . ?
YES/NO/DON'T KNOW
TABLETS/INJECTIONS/DON'T KNOW WHICH

4:2 What is the name of the tablets/injections?

. . . .

4:3 How often will . . . take these tablets/injections?

. . . .

4:4 Where will . . . get these from?

. . . .

4:5 For how long will . . . take these tablets/injections?
a few weeks/a few months/a year/2 years/more than 2 years

4:6 Do you think these tablets/injections should be taken (read out all alternatives before relative selects choice(s).

	YES	NO	DON'T KNOW
(a) When . . . thinks she/he needs them?	☐	☐	☐
(b) Until she/he seems better again?	☐	☐	☐
(c) When you (or other friends/ relatives) think he needs them?	☐	☐	☐
(d) As the doctor says/prescribes?	☐	☐	☐
(e) Not at all?	☐	☐	☐

4:7 Do you know of any side effects which might occur as a result of taking the tablets/injections?

. . . .

. . . .

. . . .

. . . .

SECTION 5: COURSE AND PROGNOSIS

	YES OR POSSIBLY	NO	DON'T KNOW
5:1 Do you think that . . . may have problems again?	☐	☐	☐

5:2 Which of the following are likely to make '(insert whatever relative calls condition)' worse, or bring her/his problems back?

	YES	NO	DON'T KNOW
(a) Having nothing to do?	☐	☐	☐
(b) Stressful life problems, (e.g. moving house, getting divorced)?	☐	☐	☐
(c) Being pushed and nagged by the family at home?	☐	☐	☐
(d) Not taking her/his tablets/ injections?	☐	☐	☐
(e) Anything else? (include items previously mentioned by relatives)	☐	☐	☐

5:3 Suppose . . . seemed and felt completely better and decided to stop taking the tablets/injections. What do you think would happen? (Read out all alternatives before relative selects choice(s).

	YES	NO	DON'T KNOW
(a) She/he would be better off without them?	☐	☐	☐
(b) It would make no difference to her/him?	☐	☐	☐
(c) She/he might start to get worse again after a while?	☐	☐	☐

SECTION 6: MANAGEMENT

6:1 Do you think there is anything you can do to help . . .'s '(insert whatever relative calls condition)'?

....
....
....
....

6:2 Do you think there is anything you should not do?

....
....
....

Do you think any of the following might help?

	YES	NO	DON'T KNOW
(a) Encouraging him/her to take her/his tablets or injections?	☐	☐	☐
(b) Looking after him/her by doing his/her washing, cooking etc.	☐	☐	☐
(c) Spending as much time as possible with her/him?	☐	☐	☐
(d) Encouraging her/him to gradually get back to doing things for her/himself?	☐	☐	☐
(e) Giving her/him a good push to get going?	☐	☐	☐

6:4 *N.B.* Ask only if relative has mentioned a potentially detrimental management strategy in this section *or elsewhere* in the interview:
ment strategy in this section *or elsewhere* in the interview:
You mentioned that you . . . (specify strategy) . . .
Probe: e.g. Could you tell me more about this?
How would you go about doing this?

References

Barrowclough, C., Tarrier, N., Watts, S., Vaughn, C., Bamrah, J.S., Freeman, H.L. (1987) Assessing the functional value of relatives' knowledge about schizophrenia. A preliminary report. *British J. Psychiatry*, 151, 1–8.

Knowledge About Schizophrenia Interview (KASI) Scoring Criteria

Each of the six sections is scored on a 4-point scale (1–4).

SECTION 1: DIAGNOSIS

Comments	Scoring Criteria	Score
	As Score '2' AND/OR gives other information which is 'incorrect' eg. 'It's not a mental illness, it's just his/her personality'.	1
	Does not know the name of the diagnosis (ie. Schizophrenia) and/or one or more answers to 1:4 incorrect according to criteria below.	2
	Knows that the name of the problem/diagnosis is Schizophrenia and that Schizophrenia is a 'severe' mental illness . . .' or at least not a minor problem. ie. In question 1:4 (a) = No, 1:4 (b) = Yes or Don't know.	3
	As score '3' and spontaneously gives additional 'correct' information e.g., names key symptoms, gives 'correct' information regarding aetiology.	4

SECTION 2: SYMPTOMATOLOGY

Scoring Criteria	**Score**
Below criteria for score '2'.	1
Meets criteria for score '3' on all questions *except* 2:5 and/or 2:2: and/or gives 'Don't Know' response to items in 2:1 and/or 2:3.	2

Must meet criteria on all questions 2:1−2:5 to score 3

{ 2:1 *At least 60%* of 'symptoms' which the relative referred to in the Camberwell Family Interview or RAI are attributed to the illness; and *none of the 'experiential' symptoms** (ie. *Delusions, hallucinations, thought problems such as broadcast, echo) are attributed to the person's natural self.
Necessary to meet criteria on questions 2:1 to 2:5.

Include her 'talking to self' and other descriptions of behaviours or beliefs which would seem to be directly associated with 'experiential' symptoms, e.g., 'suspicious ideas' } 3

Must meet criteria on all questions 2:1−2:5 to score 3

{ 2:2: Aware of at least one of the** experiential symptoms that the patient has experienced (acceptable to have mentioned one such in 2:1 or elsewhere in the interview).

**NB: Broad definition of what might be included as an experiential symptom (see *above) only applies if this corresponds with recognition of the symptom in 2:5, e.g., the relative describes a symptom of 'talking to self' on C.F.I./RAI or in 2:2 or elsewhere and recognises 'hallucinations' in 2:5, as a common and important symptom.

2:3 The patient is unable to help/ control at least 60% of 'symptoms'; and the patient is unable to help/ control all* experiential symptoms. } 3

Scoring Criteria	Score
2:4 'correct' information elicited here (e.g. delusions, hallucinations, throught problems) would be taken into consideration for score of '4' but a response to 2:4 is unnecessary for score '3'.	4
2:5 Replies 'yes' to at least 2 of the symptoms.	
Meets criteria for score '3' and gives additional information which is relevant and correct, e.g., in section 2:4.	

SECTION 3: AETIOLOGY

Scoring Criteria	Score
Necessary to ask questions 3:4*** and the response indicates that the relative will/may take action which may be detrimental to the patient, e.g., relative believes cause is a vitamin deficiency and says will encourage patient to stop medication and take vitamin supplements instead; or relative believes cause is due to the patient having an unhappy childhood and believes best 'cure' is for the relative to compensate by actions which may be over-protective.	1
***Acceptable response to questions 3:1 and 3:3 include: biological or biochemical causes; mental illness; stress or stressful life events or examples of such; e.g., stopping medication; hereditary factors.	
Necessary to ask question 3:4*** but relative's response does not indicate that the relative will take action which may be potentially detrimental to the patient and/or: 'don't know' to question 3:1 *and* 'don't know' or 'No' response to questions 3:2 (a) and/or yes to (b) and/or (c).	2

Scoring Criteria	Score
Unnecessary to ask question 3:4*** *and* all answers to questions 3:2 'correct' (3:2 (a) = yes (b) = No (c) = Yes) *AND* any answers to question 3:1 and 3:3 within acceptable 'correct' criteria or response of 'Don't Know'.	3
Meets criteria for score of '3', and gives additional 'correct' information in Questions 3:1 or 3:3, or 3:2 (d) or elsewhere, e.g., elaborates on biochemical theory.	4

SECTION 4: MEDICATION

Scoring Criteria	Score
'Incorrect' responses to questions 4:5 and/or 4:6 (or elsewhere in the interview) or don't know.	1
'Correct' responses to questions 4:5 and 4:6 (or elsewhere in the interview). Incorrect response(s) or don't know to questions 4:1 and/or 4:3 and/or 4:4.	2
Acceptable responses to questions 4:1, 4:3, 4:4 and 4:5. Correct responses to all of 4:6 (a = No, b = No, c = No, d = Yes, e = No). Answers to questions 4:2 and 4:7 need not be known.	3
As '3' with additional 'correct' information given e.g., in response to 4:2 and/or 4:7 e.g., gives two common side-effects.	4

SECTION 5: COURSE AND PROGNOSIS

Scoring Criteria	Score
'Incorrect' or 'Don't Know' response(s) to items 5:2 (c) or 5:2 (d) or any item in 5:3.	1

Scoring Criteria	Score
Item 5:2 (c) = 'correct' (Yes) or 'don't know'. Item 5:2 (d) 'correct' (Yes) and all answers to 5:3 'correct' (a) = No, (b) = No, (c) = Yes. Other responses to items may be 'incorrect' or 'don't know'.	2
Questions 5:1 = 'Yes or Possibly' (an exception is made in the case of first episode patients, when a relative's response of 'don't know' would be acceptable) *AND*	3
all answers to 5:2 'correct' (a) = Yes, (b) = Yes, (c) = Yes, (d) = Yes *AND*	
No 'incorrect' information in response to 5:2 (e) *AND* Question 5:3, all responses 'correct'.	
As for score '3' with additional 'correct' information, e.g., in question 5:2 (e).	4

SECTION 6: MANAGEMENT

Scoring Criteria	Score
Management strategies which potentially might be detrimental to the patient are mentioned in response to questions 6:1 or 6:2, or the prompts in 6:3 or 6:4 or elsewhere in the interview *AND* the relative supplies some evidence that they might be carried out. 'Potentially detrimental' would include here: arguing and quarrelling/criticising/or emotionally overinvolved behaviours.	1
As 'score 1' above, but the relative supplies no evidence that the strategies will be acted upon.	2
Acceptable responses to the prompts in 6:3, e.g.	
(a) 'Yes'; or if 'No' evidence that this is because relative wishes to avoid arguments, over-instrusive behaviour, etc.	

Scoring Criteria	Score

(b) 'No' or if 'Yes' evidence that the relative DOES NOT intend to be overprotective or to foster dependence. It is sometimes the case that, for example, a spouse will feel it might be helpful to do more of the housework following their partner's discharge. This may be beneficial to the patient. — 3

(c) 'No' or if 'Yes' evidence that the relative does not intend to spend an excessive amount of time with the patient. Each case needs to be assessed individually, but excessive might refer to: relative giving up own interests to spend time with patient/relative fearing to go out and leave patient by him/herself.

AND

No potentially detrimental management strategies (see earlier) mentioned in response to questions 6:1 and 6:2 (or elsewhere in interview).

As for score '3' *AND* 'potentially useful' strategies suggested in Section 6 or elsewhere in the interview. Such strategies might include, e.g., recognition that quarrels and criticism are not helpful but that other strategies can help, distracting patient, encouraging positive behaviours in patient, discussing problems, etc.

NB – Required to suggest an alternative strategy to score '4'.

Appendix 6

Information About Schizophrenia for Friends and Relatives

WHAT IS SCHIZOPHRENIA?

Schizophrenia is a word just about everyone has heard. Most people are not sure what schizophrenia really is, what causes it, and what can be done for it.

WHAT DO YOU UNDERSTAND BY THE TERM SCHIZOPHRENIA?

There are a few things that are definitely not schizophrenia which need to be cleared up. First, there is the common idea that schizophrenia means having more than one personality or a split personality. This is not schizophrenia. Schizophrenia means that a person finds it difficult to decide what is real and what is not real. It is a bit like having dreams when you are wide awake.

Schizophrenia is like dreaming when you are wide awake.

At times a person who has schizophrenia may act in a strange or odd manner. At other times he or she will behave in quite a reasonable way. It is often thought that people with mental illness are violent and dangerous. Usually this is not true. People suffering from schizophrenia rarely have violent outbursts, but more often they are quiet, shy and fearful.

People suffering from schizophrenia are NOT usually violent.

WHAT, THEN, IS SCHIZOPHRENIA?

Schizophrenia is a major illness. It affects about one person in every hundred in all countries throughout the world. More hospital beds are filled by people suffering from schizophrenia than from any other single illness.

One in every hundred people develops schizophrenia.

It can affect a person's everyday life in many ways, although the symptoms of schizophrenia are not the same for every person. The person's thinking may be muddled and confused. This means that they may have trouble handling everyday problems.

Schizophrenia can affect all aspects of a person's life.

He or she may not be able to work as well as before; it may be hard to concentrate and to think quickly and clearly. He or she may have similar problems with other activities. The person may find it difficult to make conversation or to show feeling, and this can make it hard to get on with people. At times the person may be so taken up with his thoughts and feelings that he or she fails to take care of even his most basic needs like sleep, food and cleanliness.

HOW DO WE KNOW WHEN A PERSON HAS SCHIZOPHRENIA?

Doctors diagnose schizophrenia when a person has certain key symptoms. They find out that the person has these symptoms mainly from what the patient tells them. Psychiatrists cannot read people's minds. There are no special blood tests or x-rays to help either. They can only make a diagnosis from what they are told. These symptoms include what are termed the Positive and Negative symptoms of schizophrenia.

Positive Symptoms

Positive symptoms are the type of symptoms that the person experiences, these are changes and distortions in their perceptions and thought processes. These type of symptoms include:

Disturbances of thinking

Thoughts being put into your head which are not your own thoughts. They may seems to come from other people by telepathy or radio waves, laser beams and so on.

Thoughts leaving your head, as if they are being taken out by somebody. Your mind is quite blank and you are unable to think about anything. This is not the same as when you forget a thought, or when you are nervous and seem to lose track of your thoughts.

Thoughts seeming to be spoken out loud as if somebody close by could hear them. Sometimes feeling that the thoughts are being broadcast from your head. In this way everybody knows what you are thinking and none of your thoughts are private.

Thought processes which become so jumbled that the person does not think in a coherent manner. This is reflected in the person's speech in which the grammar may become grossly distorted, or there are dramatic and unexpected changes from topic to topic or there is a lack of logical connection between one part of a sentence or another. Sometimes the person's speech may include made up words.

Delusions

Another disturbance of thinking is called a 'delusion'. This is a false belief that seems quite real to the person with schizophrenia. Other people do not share this belief or idea. Some examples of these delusions common in schizophrenia are:

- A belief that some other person or force has control of your thoughts or actions. That you are a zombie with no free will and another person has taken over your brain or body.

- A belief that somebody is trying to harm you, perhaps trying to kill you for no good reason. You are being unjustly persecuted.

- A belief that things that you see or read about have a special message for you. For example, seeing a red car may mean that the world is about to end.

- A belief that you are a special person or have abilities or magical powers. For example, that you are a king or a queen, or that you can cause earthquakes, floods or other natural disasters.

A delusion is a totally false belief others do not share.

These ideas often come on quite suddenly. They are unusual so that friends and family realise that they are unlikely to be really true. When the person has recovered he may be surprised what he believed when ill. It is a little like waking up from a dream.

Hallucinations

Some people have a symptom called an 'hallucination'. An hallucination is a false perception. This means that the person hears things, see things or smells things that are not heard, seen or smelt by other people. It is a little like having a dream when you are wide awake. Hearing voices when nobody is in the room is a very common symptom of schizophrenia. The voices seem real and may appear to come from the next room or outside. Sometimes they may seem to come from inside a person's head or, less often, from a part of his body. Sometimes the person believes that someone or something is touching them when there is no-one there and nothing to explain this.

An hallucination is hearing, seeing, smelling something that others do not hear, see or smell.

A diagnosis of schizophrenia is usually made because certain key positive symptoms appear to be present. However, other symptoms which are termed negative symptoms are often present at sometime during the illness.

Negative Symptoms

Unlike positive symptoms, which are dramatic changes in the person's experience, the negative symptoms are usually apparent as changes in the person's behaviour. They are termed negative because they indicate decreases or absences of behaviour. These type of symptoms include:

- An absence of motivation or enthusiasm to do anything.

- A general inactivity and a decrease in all activity levels. This may range from hobbies and leisure pursuits to simple and basic self-care activities such as washing and grooming.

- An inability to show any emotion, the person can appear flat or disinterested.

- An inability to enjoy activities that used to give pleasure.

- An apparent disinterest in conversation and talking. The person will not start conversations and frequently answer in single words if at all.

- An apparent difficulty in getting on with people even close relatives, so that contact with others will be avoided.

These negative symptoms can be very distressing for relatives, even more so than the positive symptoms. This is because all life can appear to go out of the person so that nothing interests them and they become cold and withdrawn. Many relatives also feel the person is being lazy or hurtful.

It is important to remember that these negative symptoms are part of the illness and not the person being lazy or hurtful.

Other symptoms of schizophrenia

Language difficulties
At times people suffering from schizophrenia will talk in a way that is hard to follow. Occasionally people will make up words or use odd expressions. Sometimes they may speak very little and be almost impossible to talk to.

Odd habits
These may include standing or sitting in unusual ways, peculiar manner-isms or habits.

Changed feelings and emotions
Sometimes people suffering from schizophrenia seem to show little or no feelings. At other times they may laugh or cry when they are not feeling happy or sad. Or, a person may not show normal affection for their family and friends.

Unusual Behaviour in Schizophrenia
Problems in speaking
Odd habits
Changed feelings

WHAT USUALLY HAPPENS TO PEOPLE WITH SCHIZOPHRENIA?

Schizophrenia is an illness that usually begins when a person is in their early twenties, but, it may occur at any time in a person's life. A number of people suffer only one episode of the illness and never have a further attack. But many sufferers will have periods when the symptoms return. These periods are called relapses. A few sufferers will have some symptoms all the time. For many schizophrenia is a life long concern. However, with improved medical treatment the outlook for schizophrenia is better than it has been in past years.

Schizophrenia is often a recurring illness.

Schizophrenia affects many young people in the prime of their lives. It is a major setback in their plans and hopes for the future. As a result, it is not uncommon for a person to become depressed.

WHAT CAUSES SCHIZOPHRENIA?

Schizophrenia is probably caused by a disturbance in the working of the brain. Since the illness often occurs when the person is under stress, it is thought that stress may act as a trigger to bring on the illness.

It is not exactly clear what goes wrong when a person develops schizophrenia, but it seems that chemicals in the brain are affected. This produces the symptoms of hallucinations, delusions and thinking difficulties.

We also know that taking certain types of medication improves the symptoms of schizophrenia. The medication is of course made up of chemicals. It is thought that these help to balance the chemicals in the brain.

Schizophrenia is a disorder of the brain that may be brought on by stress.

But, many scientists have studied the problem and they have not found the exact cause. At present, we still do not know what exactly causes schizophrenia. Nor do we have a total cure. We do, however, have treatment that can help people to get better.

What exactly goes wrong with the chemicals in the brain is not clear.

Is Schizophrenia a Family Illness?

Schizophrenia is an illness that can be inherited. That does not mean that if somebody in your family has the illness everybody else will get it. Nor does it mean that a person with schizophrenia should not marry and have children. We said before that people in general have about a 1 in 100 chance of getting the illness, but, if a close relative like a parent or brother or sister suffers from schizophrenia then your chances of getting the illness are higher.

It is not the illness itself that is inherited but the tendency to get it. This tendency may only develop into schizophrenia when the person is under stress. But the amount of stress it takes to bring on the illness seems to vary.

The risk of developing schizophrenia is greater if you have a parent or a brother or sister who has had the illness.

Stress and Schizophrenia

One of the greatest periods of stress, especially for young men, is in early adult life. At this time they are striving to get a good job, make friends and become independent. This is the most common time for schizophrenia to begin in men. In women, major life stress often starts later, when they have children. We find that the age at which schizophrenia tends to start is later in women.

Major stressful events such as a death in the family, loss of a job or breakup of a relationship can make schizophrenia worse or trigger off a relapse of symptoms.

Once a person has schizophrenia, the environment in which he or she lives – his family, work and so on, can help him a lot. People can support him by encouraging him to slowly regain his former skills. If they tend to push him, or nag and criticise him this may make things worse. On the other hand, if too much is done for him and he does nothing, this too can make him worse. Of course, it is impossible to totally avoid stress. But family members can help one another to cope with difficulties by taking things step by step.

Relapses may be triggered by:
1. Stressful events
2. Tension at home and work

It is clear that the family can be very helpful. But occasionally they can make things more stressful. However, there is no evidence that families cause schizophrenia.

A few years ago, many psychiatrists believed that schizophrenia was entirely caused by the way the parents brought up their children. While we all know how important this is, there is no scientific evidence that poor child care or an unhappy childhood causes schizophrenia.

Families do not cause schizophrenia.

MEDICATION

Medication was introduced for the treatment of schizophrenia about 30 years ago. It is the main form of treatment. There are several different types of drugs used in the treatment of schizophrenia, with different brand names. Medication may be given in the form of tablets or injections. Injections are often helpful as they are less likely to be forgotten. All the different types of medication have the same helpful effects.

There are two ways in which medication is used in the treatment of schizophrenia.

1. To reduce the symptoms of an attack of the illness.
2. Once the symptoms have improved, the same medication is used to prevent further attacks or the symptoms getting worse.

If the person with schizophrenia stops taking his or her medication against the doctor's advice the chances of them having a further attack of schizophrenia are more than doubled. This is why it is important to take the medication that the doctor prescribes even when the person feels completely well.

Taking medication helps to prevent relapse

Unfortunately the medication used for the treatment of schizophrenia can sometimes produce unwanted side effects. These are not usually serious and should be discussed with your doctor. Some of these side effects include drowsiness, shakiness, restlessness, and muscle stiffness. Others are sensitivity to sunburn, increased appetite, and dizziness especially when standing up suddenly.

Some of these effects the person can avoid him or herself. For example, by avoiding too much sun, by standing up slowly and watching their diet. But if your relative is worried about anything to do with the medication, go and see your doctor.

Discuss any medication worries with your doctor.

HOW CAN RELATIVES OR THE FAMILY HELP?

1. Relatives can encourage the person to take the medication that your doctor or psychiatrist has prescribed.

   Often people feel they do not need medication, especially if they are feeling well again. But it is important to take the tablets or go for the injections as they have been prescribed. The relatives can play an important role here in encouraging the patient to do this. Sometimes when the person is feeling better, he or she does not see the need to take further tablets or injections. But, if medication is stopped, a relapse may occur sooner or later. Sometimes the medication will produce side effects, these should be discussed with the doctor.

   Encourage your relative to take the medication.

2. The person with schizophrenia can be very sensitive to stress or change. Relatives can help the patient by trying to reduce stressful events or by helping the person cope with stress.

   (a) The person can be stressed by dramatic changes in routine or lifestyle, eg., moving house, or a member of the family leaving home. Where such events cannot be avoided, try to give the person advance notice. Explain the situation clearly so that any problems can be solved. Try to make any changes as gradual as possible.

   (b) If the person becomes anxious or worried, even by trivial things, encourage him/her to relax. Be patient with them and try to calm the situation down. Try not to get over concerned or upset yourself.

   You can best help the person with schizophrenia if you are calm and relaxed yourself.

   (c) Sometimes the person may become depressed and fed up. This is always difficult to cope with. Try to be sympathetic and give support. Do not blame the person, it is not their fault. Try to be encouraging and positive so that you build up a person's confidence. This can be very tiring so you both may need time away from each other. Fortunately, depression is usually only short lived.

3. Living with a person with schizophrenia can be very difficult.

   (a) They may behave in a strange way. They may spend all day in bed or take hours to get things done. They may seem not to care about themselves or others.

It is very easy to get angry or impatient especially if the person appears lazy or unhelpful. This is not surprising but it is not helpful to the person. Try to be patient and encourage gradual change. Try not to criticise or punish the person for doing things you disapprove of. This is being negative. Encourage the patient to try and praise his or her efforts. This is being positive.

Try to praise and encourage and avoid criticism and arguments.

(b) You may feel very worried. You may find you are always wondering what will happen next and how you will cope. The best thing is not to spend too much time together. Try not to be too fussy or over protective. It is important that the person is encouraged to lead an independent life and gain confidence in him or herself.

Encourage the person to gradually become more independent and confident.

(c) You may find that you become anxious or depressed yourself. Try to relax. It is often helpful to talk over your feelings with someone else. Try to keep your own interest and hobbies going. You need time for yourself and this will take your mind off things. Getting very worried and overconcerned can make things worse.

If a crisis occurs, do not feel guilty or blame yourself. You cannot anticipate everything. Try to cope with situations as calmly as possible as they arise. Try not to over-react and try to stay relaxed. Sometimes there are no right answers, but learning comes from experience.

Make time for yourself. This will help everyone.

4. Family Problem Solving

Living with someone who suffers from schizophrenia can cause tensions at home. It can increase the impact of other problems.

Sometimes it may be useful to get the family together to talk things out. Be clear about what the problem is. Allow everyone to express their views and feelings. Listen to one another but try not to argue or criticise. Try to find different ways of dealing with the problem. Agree together on the best thing to do and how to carry it out. This is a positive approach to solving problems. It stops wasting time arguing and being negative.

Talk things over. Try to find solutions together.

FAMILIES DO NOT CAUSE SCHIZOPHRENIA

SUMMARY

1. Schizophrenia is a major mental illness that affects 1 in 100 people.
2. The symptoms include delusions–false beliefs; hallucinations–false perceptions, usually voices; difficulties of thinking, feelings and behaviour.
3. The exact cause is not known but there appears to be an inbalance of the brain chemistry.
4. Stress and tension make the symptoms worse and possibly trigger the illness.
5. People who develop schizophrenia possibly have a tendency which may run in families. This increases their risk of getting schizophrenia.
6. Some people recover from schizophrenia completely, but most have some difficulties and may suffer relapses.
7. Although there are no complete cures available, relapses can be prevented and life difficulties overcome.
8. It is VERY important to take the medication prescribed.
9. Family members and friends can be most helpful by:
   - Encouraging the person to take the medication
   - Staying calm and relaxed themselves
   - Being encouraging and positive
   - Solving family problems in a calm way

Guidelines for Evaluating Relatives' Beliefs; Key Issues to be Targeted During Sessions; Common Themes, Questions, and Concerns Raised by Relatives in Information-Giving Sessions

THE DIAGNOSIS

Helpful Information

It is useful for the relatives to know the name of the diagnosis. Although we acknowledge the harmful effects of labelling, and that some relatives might be fearful or distressed by the word 'schizophrenia', there are a number of reasons why it is helpful for the relative to be aware of the terminology: knowing the name gives them access to support groups – principally the Schizophrenia Fellowship, in the UK – and information about schizophrenia; if they do not hear the term from you or medical staff, they may be exposed to the diagnosis in a situation where support and education is unavailable – several relatives and patients reported first learning of the diagnosis from sickness benefit notes or overheard conversations; relatives and patients have a right to share the information which is available to medical staff.

Unhelpful Information

Although we feel that knowing the term 'schizophrenia' can be potentially useful to the relative, it is the belief that the patient has an alternative condition rather than just not knowing the diagnosis that can be potentially unhelpful, since this belief could lead to management strategies that may be detrimental to the illness course. An extreme example was a husband who denied his wife had a mental illness and who believed she had a vitamin deficiency: his management strategy was to discourage her taking medication and to closely supervise her diet! Other less extreme examples are relatives who attribute the patient's condition to street drugs or alcohol, or personality problems, rather than to mental illness. Some of problems with such beliefs are that the patient may be seen to have more control over their problems than is true for schizophrenia, and that continuing to take medication is unnecessary or possibly harmful.

Common Themes, Questions, and Concerns

'My GP said she had a psychosis, not schizophrenia.' 'The other hospital said it was a nervous breakdown.'
Such comments can be discussed in terms of there being many general names for the kind of symptoms the patient has experienced. The word 'schizophrenia' does not contradict the other descriptions of the patient's problems, but the term 'schizophrenia' is used when a person has certain key symptoms, (which you will go on to discuss). Knowing the medical diagnosis may be helpful to the relative for understanding the kinds of problems and treatments the patient will receive. There is no reason, however, why the relative should not continue to use an alternative description, and terms such as 'breakdown' or even 'psychosis' might be easier for communicating with friends or relatives, since, unfortunately, many people are fearful of the term 'schizophrenia', and the patient could be stigmatized or rejected.

'I don't think it is schizophrenia; he's not like the really disturbed cases you see on TV' 'She's not violent – she can't be schizophrenic'.
Violence in schizophrenia is often an issue for relatives in education sessions. Before having someone in the family with the illness, most people's experience of the word is associated with characters in books or films who commit bizarre crimes and murders. Thus the fact that the patient has shown no evidence of physical aggression may be given as a reason for rejecting the diagnosis, or relatives may be fearful that the patient could become violent. An emphasis on the unfairness of the media in perpetuating myths of violent behaviours, and some statement of the evidence that people suffering from the illness are more likely to be shy and fearful is usually sufficient to allay people's fears. However, some schizophrenic patients do become violent under some circumstances (Chapter 9).

THE SYMPTOMS

Helpful Information

It is useful for relatives to understand that the key symptoms experienced when people with schizophrenia are acutely ill cannot be seen directly, but rather are thoughts, ideas, and voices that go on inside the person's head. This understanding is important for helping the relative to work out why the patient has behaved/is behaving strangely.

Although the patient may not have discussed these experiences with the relative, the relative may have some understanding through seeing the patient behave strangely: 'as if' talking to someone when no one is there; giggling to oneself; seeming afraid or hiding indoors; becoming alarmed when the TV or radio is on, and so on. The education session should help the relative to understand the nature of the positive symptoms which have directed the patient's behaviour. A recognition that the experiential symptoms are real to the patient is the aim, since this may help the relative to understand that the patient cannot easily control his/her disturbed behaviours: resist answering the voices; be dissuaded from fears; watch the TV without alarm.

An understanding of the psychopathology of schizophrenia as a whole need not be given too much emphasis, unless the relative is particularly interested in acquiring such academic knowledge. It is important to give some emphasis to the negative symptoms of schizophrenia, and again, where appropriate, to give concrete examples from the patient's behaviour and to stress that negative symptoms cannot easily be overcome by the patient.

Unhelpful Information

Relatives' beliefs that problem-patient behaviours arise largely from personality traits or could be controlled if the patient were willing to make more effort, need to be targeted for change during the information sessions. That is not to say that the relative needs to be of the opinion that all of the problems are outside of the patient's control: there is sometimes the danger that an overemphasis on lack of control and illness concepts will lead the relative to wrap the patient in cotton wool, or to feel guilty if they make small demands on them.

We are particularly concerned that the relative is aware of the positive symptoms which have directed or continue to direct the patient's disturbed behaviour, and that some of the difficulties for the patient in getting on with ordinary tasks of living may be caused by the negative illness symptoms, and that such symptoms and difficulties can only be controlled by the patient with exceptional effort, or not at all.

Common Themes, Questions, and Concerns

'She's never heard voices, I don't think that's a symptom'
Relatives often find it difficult to focus on the symptoms of schizophrenia
in general, and will repeatedly return to the specific experience of illness
in their son/daughter/husband/wife. This is not usually a problem,
but it is worthwhile informing the relative that each patient's symptom
pattern is different, but the same patient can have different symptoms on
different occasions of illness. If the patient in question has not had
hallucinations, then no doubt the relative will pay little attention to the
idea that hallucinations are a diagnostic symptom. But if the patient
relapses at some future date and does hallucinate, then the relative may
recall the information from an education session and find it useful in
understanding the patient's behaviour.

*'You say that lying on the settee a lot is caused by illness symptoms. How is it
that he can do things that he wants to, like going to the pub, but can't be bothered
to help in the house?'*
This theme recurs in relatives, and if not brought up in the initial
information sessions may well become an issue during later meetings.
Essentially, it is very difficult for relatives to grasp the idea that deficits in
activities of ordinary living can be attributed to an illness which has no
other physical manifestations. The logic of the relative's thinking is clear:
if the person's illness makes them lethargic, then this lethargy should be
seen in all their behaviour, not just selected aspects. It is important to
address the issue raised with some understanding: you see they have a
point, and you are glad they have given you an example. Perhaps the fact
that the patient can go to the pub tells you something about how he/she
can be helped to do other activities, and this will be useful when you go
on to look at ways in which you work together to improve the patient's
recovery. What's different for the patient in going to the pub that is not
the case with doing the washing-up, or some other specific household
task? What does the patient get out of going to the pub that he does not
get from doing the washing-up? This kind of prompting will sometimes
lead the relative to come up with factors which differentiate the two
situations: the patient always liked/felt comfortable/more relaxed from
drinking in the pub/a friend calls round to go to the pub with him/he
(and most people) did not get much pleasure/reward from washing-up.

The therapist can offer such suggestions if they are not spontaneously
mentioned, and go on to emphasize that negative symtoms do not mean
that the person is unable to perform activities; rather that activities
require exceptional effort on the part of the patient and normal pleasure
or satisfaction from doing things is much diminished, thus the patient is

more likely to perform tasks if they have strong intrinsic rewards. Much of the effort is required to start a task, and once thay have begun, continuing can be easier. Analogies can be made of how people behave when they are feeling weak when recovering from an illness: if a friend comes round to see them, the person may rally round and get out of bed to make the visitor a cup of tea and feel that the effort required is worth it if they enjoy the friend's company, but without the visit they would have preferred to stay in bed. In a similar way, encouraging the patient to begin doing more by focusing on previously enjoyed activities and giving them help and encouragement in the early stages can be good strategies for rehabilitating the patient at home.

AETIOLOGY

Helpful Information

Most relatives will have given considerable thought to 'why' questions about the reasons for the patient getting ill. While the absence of any explanation is unusual, the relative who has not already come up with a causative theory is not at a disadvantage, since they will often take on board the explanations offered to them much more readily than a relative who has developed their own causative model. Relatives who have or who are able to assimilate causal models whereby stress and biological factors are important will find these concepts useful in helping to manage the illness: they will have the bones of the rationale for interventions that seek to reduce stress and adhere to prophylactic medications. An idea that stress can be both long term and cumulative – as in the case of problematic relationships at home – as well as from one-off events (both good and bad) is also useful for setting the scene for further work with the family.

Unhelpful Information

Theories of aetiology which do not fit in with the limited knowledge we have about the causes of schizophrenic illness are best judged in terms of their likely consequences for the relative's management of the illness at home. Thus the belief that the illness was caused by the patient's own behaviour – smoking marijuana, drinking too much alcohol, being 'too sensitive', having 'too big an imagination' – are not harmful in themselves, but become problematic if the relative acts upon such beliefs as being the sole causal agents in the illness. This might involve attempting to stop access to street drugs or alcohol through coercion, or trying to talk the patient out of delusional ideas, or protect them from stress by over-involved behaviours. In both cases, this means not accepting the legitimacy of symptoms, the need to reduce household stress, or the need for long-term medication. Theories which invoke the relatives' own causal role in the onset of the illness, for example, the idea that they have let the patient down in some way and this has precipitated the illness, or could have averted the illness if they had given the patient more attention, can be problematic since they can make the relative feel guilty and depressed.

Common Themes, Questions, and Concerns

'You say that alcohol [or marijuana] doesn't cause schizophrenia. Why is it then that she has always been drinking a lot when she gets ill?'
The association between drink or other substance abuse and relapse is often raised by relatives. It may sometimes be the case that drink or drugs are used by patients to reduce the increased anxiety or arousal levels that they experience preceding or during a schizophrenic episode, and this can be offered as an alternative explanation of why relapse and drinking or drugs often go together. Relatives may be worried that even if drink/drugs do not cause schizophrenia, they may have adverse effects e.g., interfere with the action of the prescribed medication, and this point is quite valid, particularly if the patient is drinking or smoking marijuana to excess. Each case needs to be assessed, and there are no general answers. It is often best dealt with at this stage by acknowledging that the problem should be addressed, and putting it on the agenda for a future session. The difficulty is that substance abuse is often the focus of arguments between the patient and his relatives, and alternative strategies for reducing the problem need to be implemented, rather than the relative increasing their attempts to coerce the patient into stopping drinking/taking drugs.

'Can he/she have children, and would they be likely to have schizophrenia?'
This question may be prompted by giving relatives some information on the genetic contribution to schizophrenia. The simple answers are: yes he/she can have children, i.e., schizophrenia in itself does not prevent one having a sexual relationship or from becoming pregnant, and, no, any offspring would be more likely not to develop schizophrenia than to have the illness. The risk of having the illness, however, is increased when there is a close blood relative in the family who has the illness. The risks range from 1% in the general population through to 3% for grandchildren, nephews/nieces, and 10% for siblings or offspring.

Such answers can be moderated by explaining that the tendency to develop the illness is in some cases inherited, but that the illness often only develops under stress, and that the amount and kind of stress it takes to bring on the illness varies from person to person. This individual 'stress/diathesis' model can be best explained in terms of an analogy. A talent or skill, such as being a good football player, or musician or mathematician, is a useful one. Some people could become good footballers if they were given a lot of intensive coaching and encouragement; others would shine at football without any encouragement; and some would be hopeless players no matter how much help they got. In the same way, some people with an inherited tendency would only develop schizophrenia if they had a massive amount of stress over a prolonged period; some people with the inherited tendency would develop the illness with little or no stress; and some people do not have the inherited tendency, and thus could not develop schizophrenia no matter how much stress they had.

MEDICATION

Helpful Information

Using our criteria of what information is useful to the relative in the management of the illness, it is helpful for the relative to understand that the medication will need to be taken for a long period, if not indefinitely, and that it should not be terminated when the patient seems to be better. These facts will help the relative to encourage compliance, as will the practical details of where the patient will obtain medications, and with what frequency injections will be needed or pills prescribed. Some knowledge of common, unwanted, and preventable side effects of neuroleptic medication is of obvious value.

Unhelpful Information

Failure to encourage the patient to adhere to prescribed medication, or worse, the active dissuasion of the patient to have prescribed injections and pills may arise from ignorance of their role both in treatment and relapse prevention. Sometimes the relative believes that the medication acts like minor tranquilizers and is helpful to calm the patient down in the short term but may become 'addictive" with prolonged use, and it is better for the patient to learn to cope without medication since they may otherwise become dependent on the tranquilizing effects.

Common Themes, Questions, and Concerns

'What about the harmful effects of the drugs? Is it worth the risks to take them for life?'
Rather than taking a dogmatic line about adherence to prescribed medication, questions like this can usefully be approached by encouraging patients and relatives to assess the pros and cons of medication, and to

add up both sides of the argument. On the pro side, there are the benefits of reduced relapse risks; some 'immunity' to life stresses; and improved ability to function normally through the reduction in positive symptoms. On the cons side, there are the possible side-effects, and sometimes a general dislike of the idea of prolonged dependence on medication.

Reassurance about how side-effects can be eliminated by using additional drugs, and by changing or reducing medications, and by taking simple precautions, as with sensitivity to sun exposure, can be helpful. The idea of long-term medication management of illnesses can be somewhat 'normalized' by introducing analogies with physical conditions which require prophylactic medicine, such as diabetes. The diabetic analogy is particularly useful: in both diabetes and schiziophrenia the medications compensate, at least partially, for a biochemical abnormality. Their action is not a cure, and the underlying abnormality is still present, hence the need for continued and long-term use of drugs to prevent symptoms recurring.

'What do the drugs do?'
Answers to this question will depend on the level of explanation that the relative is pursuing and is able to understand. It is useful for the therapist to familiarize themselves with the theory that antipsychotic drugs act by blocking dopamine receptors, and a few patients and relatives have requested more detailed references on the subject (Further Reading). Usually, an explanation along the lines that schizophrenia develops from a malfunctioning of the brain, that antipsychotic drugs work by compensating for the brain malfunction, and that this involves restoring a chemical inbalance, the result being the patient experiences less hallucinations, delusions, and faulty thinking, is sufficient.

'The newspapers and TV are full of advice against taking tranquillizers.'
Relatives are often understandably confused about the role of medication in psychiatric problems, given the emphasis on alternative medicines and the publicity that the harmful long-term consequences of taking minor tranquillizers has received. Also the term 'major tranquillizers' can be misleading and is best avoided: it sounds as if antipsychotic medication is a bigger or more powerful dose of minor tranquillizers. When relatives are confused about the effects of minor tranquillizers and neuroleptics, or introduce the worries about the addictive properties of neuroleptics, it is useful to make a clear distinction between the two. Tranquillizers or sedatives are used to treat people with anxiety problems: their effects include a general calming or tranquillizing of stress feelings and thoughts, and a relaxing of physical tension. On the other hand, the principal action of antipsychotic medication is not to tranquillize or sedate, but specifically to reduce hallucinations and delusions.

COURSE AND PROGNOSIS

Helpful Information

It is helpful if relatives are aware that once a patient has had an episode of schizophrenia, there is a real possibility that the illness will recur. This awareness is helpful in as much as it provides a rationale for the patient taking long-term medication; and that stressful life events and environments can have a role in increasing the chances of relapse.

Unhelpful Information

Although believing that the illness is unlikely to recur may be helpful to the relative in the short term by making them feel optimistic about the future, the consequences of this line of thought may prevent them from giving the kind of support and engagement in a programme of advice that will benefit the patient. It is likely also to set them up for disappointment in the long term, and an understanding of the risks of relapse alongside an appreciation of what can be done to reduce the risks and help the patient have a reasonable quality of life is better than concealing what is known of the prognosis.

Common, Themes, Questions, and Concerns

'Will he/she ever be cured?'
A 'cure' to most relatives means that the patient will be free of all his/her symptoms and problems, will have no need of further treatment, and there will be no possibility of the illness recurring. The following can be fed back to the relative when questions about 'cures' are raised: If you mean by cure . . . then the simple answer is no, at this time there is no cure available for schizophrenia. However, the chances that a person can get over an episode of schizophrenia and resume a near normal life are often good. Among patients diagnosed as having schizophrenia there are huge differences in severity of illness and recovery of functioning.'

This kind of statement needs to be modified according to the chronicity and severity of the illness in question. For patients who have a long history of residual symptoms and low social functioning it would be more appropriate to talk about reduction in symptoms and improvements in the patient's ability to live independently. Positive aspects of the future can then be raised: antipsychotic medication can reduce or even eradicate the delusions and hallucinations and greatly reduce the risk of the symptoms recurring; rehabilitation programmes and family support can greatly assist in getting the patient back to living a normal life.

MANAGEMENT

Helpful Information

It is helpful for the relative to understand that some common ways that people try to control the behaviour of others are not helpful with a person who has a schizophrenic illness: included here are attempts to restore behaviour or stop symptoms by coercion through arguments, verbal persuasions, and threats; or attempts to make things right by doing everything for the patient, feeling unable to leave them alone or intruding in all their decision making (Chapter 4). Helpful ideas include 'constructive' strategies, such as: encouraging and prompting the patient to gradually get back to everyday activities; using shared problem solving approaches to difficulties in the family; helping the patient prepare for changes and life events; sympathizing but not colluding with delusions and using distraction techniques; encouraging the patient to take medications and to discuss compliance problems with medical staff; keeping up the relatives' own interests and not focusing their own life around the patient.

Unhelpful Information

All beliefs that coercive or controlling methods will get the patient well would be considered unhelpful; also centring their own life around that of the patient; failure to endorse medication compliance; and all strategies contrary to those listed above.

Common Themes, Questions, and Concerns

'I find that she/he won't do anything unless I really shout at him/her.'
If this kind of comment is made, it is often useful to talk about methods of dealing with problems in the short term, as opposed to strategies which make for longer-term change. While nagging or shouting may prompt a person into action on one occasion, it is often the case that the problem is only temporarily resolved. Moreover, the shouting or nagging may cause both parties some upset and distress, particularly if it continues and arguments develop.

'Before I knew he/she was ill, I used to get on at him/her a lot. Now I feel guilty.'
This sort of remark indicates that the relative needs considerable reassurance on the lines that their confusion about what was the matter with the patient was quite normal, and that they in no way could have caused the illness, or even made it worse.

References

Barrelet, L., Ferrero, F., Szigethy, *et al*. (1990) Expressed emotion and first admission schizophrenia: nine-month follow-up in a French cultural environment. *British J. Psychiatry*, 156, 357–62.

Barrowclough, C. (1991) Attributions and expressed emotion in the relatives of schizophrenic patients. Unpub. thesis, Univ. London.

Barrowclough, C. and Tarrier, N. (1984) Psychosocial interventions with families and their effects on the course of schizophrenia: a review. *Psych. Medicine*, 14, 629–42.

Barrowclough, C. and Tarrier, N. (1987) A behavioural family intervention with a schizophrenic patient: a case study. *Behavioural Psychotherapy*, 15, 252–71.

Barrowclough, C. and Tarrier, N. (1990) Social functioning in schizophrenic patients. I: The effects of expressed emotion and family intervention. *Social Psychiatry and Psychiatric Epidemiology*, 25, 125–9.

Barrowclough, C., Tarrier, N., Watts, S., *et al*. (1987) Assessing the functional value of relatives' reported knowledge about schizophrenia. *British J. Psychiatry*, 151, 1–8.

Bentall, R.P., Jackson, H.F. and Pilgrim, D. (1988) Abandoning the concept of 'schizophrenia': some implications of validity arguments for psychological research into psychotic phenomena. *British J. Clinical Psychology*, 27, 303–24.

Berkowitz, R., Eberlein-Fries, R., Kuipers, L. and Leff, J. (1984) Educating relatives about schizophrenia. *Schizophrenia Bulletin*, 7, 418–29.

Bernheim, K. (1989) Psychologists and families of the severely mentally ill: the role of family consultation. *American Psychologist*, 44, 561–4.

Birchwood, M., Smith, J., MacMillan, F., *et al*. (1989) Predicting relapse in schizophrenia: the development and implementation of an early signs monitoring system using patients and families as observers, a preliminary investigation. *Psychological Medicine*, 19, 649–56.

Birchwood, M., Smith, J., Cochrane, R., *et al*. (1990) The social functioning scale: the development and validation of a scale of social adjustment for use in family intervention programmes with schizophrenic patients. *British J. Psychiatry*, 157, 853–9.

Birchwood, M., Smith, J. and Cochrane, R. (1991) Specific and non-specific effects of educational intervention for families living with schizophrenia: a comparison of three methods. *British J. Psychiatry* (in press).

Blackburn I.M. and Davidson, K.A. (1990) *Cognitive Therapy for Depression and Anxiety*, Scientific Publications, Oxford.

Breier, A. and Strauss, J.S. (1983) Self-control in psychotic disorders. *Archives of General Psychiatry*, 40, 1141–5.

Brewin, C., MacCarthy, B., Duda, K. and Vaughan, C. (1991) Attribution and expressed emotion in the relatives of patients with schizophrenia. *J. Abnormal Psychology* (in press).

Brown, G.W. (1985) The discovery of expressed emotion: induction or deduction in *Expressed Emotion in Families*, (eds J. Leff and C. Vaughn) Guilford, New York.

Brown, G.W. and Birley, J.L.T. (1968) Crises and life changes and the onset of schizophrenia. *J. Health and Social Behaviour*, 9, 203–14.

Brown, G.W., Monck, E.M., Carstairs, *et al.* (1962) Influence of family life on the course of schizophrenic illness. *British J. Preventative Social Medicine*, 16, 55–68.

Brown, G.W., Birley, J.L.T. and Wing, J.K. (1972) Influence of family life on the course of schizophrenic disorders: a replication. *British J. Psychiatry*, 121, 241–58.

Caldwell, C.B. and Gettesman, I.I. (1990) Schizophrenics kill themselves too. *Schizophrenia Bulletin*, 16, 571–90.

Cardin, V.A., McGill, C.W. and Falloon, I.R.H. (1986) An economic analysis: Costs, benefits and effectiveness, in *Family Management of Schizophrenia*, (ed I.R.H. Falloon) John Hopkins Univ. Press, Baltimore.

Carpenter, W.T. and Heinrichs, D.W. (1983) Early intervention, time-limited, targeted pharmacotherapy of schizophrenia. *Schizophrenia Bulletin*, 9, 533–542.

Cazullo, C.L., Bertrando, P., Bressi, *et al.* (1988) Emotivita expressa e schizofrenia: studio prospettico di replicazione. *Notizie ARS*, Suppl. al. No. 3/88, 16–21.

Cheek, F.E., Laucius, J., Mahnoke, M., *et al.* (1971) A behavior modification training programme for parents of convalescent schizophrenics, in *Advances in Behavior Therapy*, Vol 3, (ed R. Rubin), Academic Press, New York.

Clements, K. and Turpin, G. (1991) Vunerability models and schizophrenia: the assessment and prediction of relapse, in *Innovations in the Psychological Management of Schizophrenia: Assessment, Treatment and Services*, (eds M. Birchwood and N. Tarrier) Wiley, Chichester.

Creer, C. and Wing, J.K. (1974) *Schizophrenia in the Home*. National Schizophrenia Fellowship, Surbiton.

Crow, T.J. (1980a) Molecular pathology: more than one disease process? *British Medical J.*, 280, 66–8.

Crow, T.J. (1980b) Positive and negative schizophrenic symptoms and the role of dopamine. *British J. Psychiatry*, 137, 383–6.

Curson, D.A., Barnes, T.R.E., Bamber, R.W., *et al.* (1985) Long-term depot maintenance of chronic schizophrenic outpatients. *British J. Psychiatry*, 146, 464–80.

Curson, D.A., Patel, M., Liddle, P.F., *et al.* (1988) Psychiatric morbidity of a long-stay hospital population with chronic schizophrenia and implications for future community care. *British Medical J.*, 297, 819–22.

Curran, J.P., Faraone, S. and Graves, D.J. (1988) Acute inpatient settings, in *Handbook of Behavioural Family Therapy*, (ed I.R.H. Falloon) Guilford Press, New York.

Dawson, M.E. and Nuechterlein, K.H. (1984) Psychophysiological dysfunctions in the developmental course of schizophrenic disorders. *Schizophrenia Bulletin*, 10, 204–32.

Dawson, M.E., Nuechterlein, K.H. and Adams, R.M. (1989) Schizophrenic disorders, in *Handbook of Clinical Psychophysiology*, (ed G. Turpin) Wiley, Chichester.

Day, R., Nielsen, J.A., Korten, A., Ernberg, *et al.* (1987) Stressful life events preceding the acute onset of schizophrenia: A cross-national study from the World Health Organisation. *Culture and Medical Psychiatry*, 11, 123–206.

De Angelis, T. (1991) Schizophrenia: Violence link disputed. *American Psychological Association Monitor*, 22, (2) Feb. 25.

Dohrenwend, B.P., Levav, I., Shrout, P.E., *et al*. (1987) Life stress and psychopathology. *American J. Community Psychology*, 15, 677–715.

Doherty, J., Van Kammen, D., Siris, S., *et al*. (1978) Stages of onset of schizophrenic psychosis. *American J. Psychiatry*, 135, 420–6.

Dulz, B. and Hand, I. (1986) Short-term relapse in young schizophrenics: can it be predicted and affected by family (CFI), patient and treatment variables? An experimental study, in *Treatment of Schizophrenia: Family Assessment and Intervention*, (eds M.J. Goldstein, I. Hand and K. Hahlweg) Springer-Verlag, Berlin.

Engel, G.L. (1977) The need for a new medical model: a challenge for biomedicine. *Science*, 196, 129–36.

Fadden, G., Kuipers, I. and Bebbington, P. (1987) The burden of care: the impact of functional psychiatric illness on the patient's family. *British J. Psychiatry*, 150, 285–92.

Falloon, I.R.H. (1986) Cognitive and behavioural interventions in the self-control of schizophrenia, in *Psychosocial Treatment of Schizophrenia: Multidimensional Concepts, Psychological, Family, and Self-Help Perspectives*, (eds J.S. Strauss, W. Boker, *et al*.) Hans Huber, Bern.

Falloon, I.R.H. (1988) Expressed emotion: current status. *Psychological Medicine*, 18, 269–74.

Falloon, I.R.H. and Pederson, J. (1985) Family management in the prevention of morbidity of schizophrenia: the adjustment of the family unit. *British J. Psychiatry*, 147, 156–63.

Falloon, I.R.H. and Talbot, R.E. (1981) Persistent auditory hallucinations: coping mechanisms and implications for management. *Psychological Medicine*, 11, 329–39.

Falloon, I.R.H., Watt, D.C. and Shepherd, M. (1978) A comparative controlled trial of pimozide and fluphenazine decanoate in the continuation therapy of schizophrenia. *Psychological Medicine*, 7, 59–70.

Falloon, I.R.H., Boyd, J.L., McGill, C.W., *et al*. (1982) Family management in the prevention of exacerbations of schizophrenia. *New England J. Medicine*, 306, 1437–40.

Falloon, I.R.H., Boyd, J.L. and McGill, C. (1984) *Family Care of Schizophrenia*. Guilford Press, New York.

Falloon, I.R.H., Boyd, J.L., McGill, C.W., *et al*. (1985) Family management in the prevention of morbidity of schizophrenia: clinical outcome of a two-year longitudinal study. *Archives of General Psychiatry*, 42, 887–96.

Flesch, R. (1948) A new readability yardstick. *J. Applied Psychology*, 32, 221–3.

Georgiades, N.J. and Phillimore, L. (1975) The myth of the hero-innovator and alternative strategies for organizational change, in *Behaviour Modification with the Severely Retarded*, (eds C.C. Kiernan and F.P. Woodford) Associated Scientific.

Goldberg, D.P. (1972) *The Detection of Psychiatric Illness by Questionnaire*. Maudsley Monograph No 21, Oxford Univ. Press, Oxford.

Goldberg, D.P. and Williams, P. (1988) *A User's Guide to the General Health Questionnaire*, NFER-Nelson, Windsor.

Goldstein, M.J. and Kopeikin, H.S. (1981) Short- and long-term effects of combining drug and family therapy, in *New Developments in Intervention with Families of Schizophrenics*, (ed M.J. Goldstein) Jossey-Bass, San Fransisco.

Goldstein, M.J. (1990) Risk factors and prevention in schizophrenia, in *Recent*

Advances in Schizophrenia, (eds A. Kales, C.N. Stefanis and J. Talbott) Springer-Verlag, New York.

Goldstein, M.J., Rodnick, E.H., Evans, J.R., *et al.* (1978) Drug and family therapy in the aftercare of acute schizophrenia. *Archives of General Psychiatry*, 35, 1169–77.

Goldstein, M.J., Miklowitz, D., Strachan, A., *et al.* (1989) Patterns of expressed emotion and patient coping styles that characterise the families of recent onset schizophrenics. *British J. Psychiatry*, 155 (Suppl. 5), 107–111.

Greenley, J.R. (1986) Self-control and expressed emotion. *J. Nervous and Mental Diseases*, 174, 24–30.

Hafner, H. and An der Heiden, W. (1989) The evaluation of mental health care systems. *British J. Psychiatry*, 155, 12–17.

Hahlweg, K., Goldstein, M.J., Nuechterlein, K.H., *et al.* (1989) Expressed Emotion and patient-relative interaction in families of recent onset schizophrenics. *J. Consulting and Clinical Psychology*, 57, 11–18.

Hawton, K., Salkovskis, P.M., Kirk, J. *et al.* (1989) *Cognitive Behaviour Therapy for Psychiatric Problems*. Oxford Univ. Press, Oxford.

Heinrichs, D.W. (1988) The treatment of delusions in schizophrenic patients, in *Delusional Beliefs*, (eds T.F. Oltmanns and B.A. Maher) Wiley, New York.

Heinrichs, D.W., Cohen, B. and Carpenter, W. (1985) Early insight and the management of schizophrenic decompensation. *J. Nervous and Mental Diseases*, 173, 133–8.

Hemsley, D. (1986) Psychological treatment of schizophrenia, in *A Handbook of Clinical Psychology*, (eds S. Lindsay and G. Powell) Gower, London.

Herz, M.I. and Melville, C. (1980) Relapse in schizophrenia. *American J. Psychiatry*, 137, 801–5.

Herz, M.I., Glazer, W.M., Mostert, M.A., *et al.* (1991) Intermittent vs maintenance medication in schizophrenia: two-year results. *Archives of General Psychiatry*, 48, 333–9.

Hirsch, S.R. and Leff, J.P. (1975) *Abnormalities in Parents of Schizophrenics*. Maudsley Monograph No 22, Oxford Univ. Press, London.

Hogarty, G., Schooler, N.R., Ulrich, R.F., *et al.* (1979) Fluphenazine and social therapy in the aftercare of schizophrenic patients. *Archives of General Psychiatry*, 36, 1283–94.

Hogarty, G., Anderson, C.M., Reiss, D.J., *et al.* (1986) Family psychoeducation, social skills training and maintenance chemotherapy in the aftercare treatment of schizophrenia. I: one-year effects of a controlled study on relapse and expressed emotion. *Archives of General Psychiatry*, 43, 633–42.

Hogarty, G., Anderson, C.M. and Reiss, D.J. (1987) Family psychoeducation, social skills training and medication in schizophrenia: the long and the short of it. *Psychopharmacological Bulletin*, 23, 12–13.

Hogarty, G., Anderson, C.M., Reiss, D.J., *et al.* (1991) Family psychoeducation, social skills training and maintenance chemotherapy in the aftercare treatment of schizophrenia. II: two-year effects of a controlled study on relapse and adjustment. *Archives of General Psychiatry*, 48, 340–47.

Hooley, J.M. (1985) Expressed emotion: a review of the critical literature. *Clinical Psychology Review*, 5, 119–39.

Hudson, B. (1975) A behaviour modification project with chronic schizophrenics in the community. *Behaviour Research and Therapy*, 13, 339–41.

Jolley, A.G., Hirsch, S.R., McRink, A., *et al.* (1989) Trial of brief intermittent neuroleptic prophylaxis for selected schizophrenic outpatients: clinical outcome at one year. *British Medical J.*, 298, 985–90.

Karno, M., Jenkins, J.H., de la Silva, A., *et al.* (1987) Expressed emotion and schizophrenic outcome among Mexican-American families. *J. Nervous and Mental Diseases*, 175, 143–51.

Kellner, R. and Sheffield, B.F. (1973) A self-rating scale of distress. *Psychological Medicine*, 3, 88–100.

Koenigsberg, H.W. and Handley, R. (1986) Expressed emotion: from predictive index to clinical construct. American J. Psychiatry, 143, 1361–73.

Kottgen, C., Soinnichsen, I., Mollenhauer, K., *et al.* (1984) Results of the Hamburg Camberwell family Interview study, I–III. *International J. Family Psychiatry*, 5, 61–94.

Krawiecka, M., Goldberg, D.P. and Vaughan, M. (1977) A standardised psychiatric assessment scale for rating chronic psychotic patients. *Acta Psychiatrica Scandinavica*, 55, 299–308.

Kuipers, L. (1979) Expressed emotion: a review. *British J. Social and Clinical Psychology*, 18, 237–44.

Kuipers, L. and Bebbington, P. (1988) Expressed emotion research in schizophrenia: theoretical and clinical implications. *Psychological Medicine*, 18, 893–909.

Leff, J. (1989) Controversial issues and growing points in research on relatives' expressed emotion. *International J. Social Psychiatry*, 35, 133–45.

Leff, J. and Vaughn, C. (1985) *Expressed Emotion in Families: its Significance for Mental Illness*. Guilford Press, New York.

Leff, J., Kuipers, L., Berkowitz, R., *et al.* (1982) A controlled trial of intervention in the families of schizophrenic families. *British J. Psychiatry*, 141, 121–34.

Leff, J., Kuipers, L., Berkowitz, R. and Sturgeon, D. (1985) A controlled trial of social intervention in the families of schizophrenic patients: two year follow-up. *British J. Psychiatry*, 146, 594–600.

Leff, J., Wig, N., Ghosh, A., *et al.* (1987) III. Influence of relatives' expressed emotion on the course of schizophrenia in Chandigarh. *British J. Psychiatry*, 151, 215–16.

Leff, J., Berkowitz, R., Shavit, A., *et al.* (1989) A trial of family therapy v. a relatives group for schizophrenia. *British J. Psychiatry*, 154, 58–66.

Leff, J., Wig, N., Ghosh, A., *et al.* (1990a) Relatives' expressed emotion and the course of schizophrenia in Chandigarh: a two-year follow-up of a first contact sample. *British J. Psychiatry*, 156, 351–6.

Leff, J., Berkowitz, R., Shavit, A., *et al.* (1990b) A trial of family therapy v. a relatives group for schizophrenia: two-year follow-up. *British J. Psychiatry*, 157, 571–7.

Lefley, H.P. (1989) Family burden and family stigma in major mental illness. *American Psychologist*, 44, 556–60.

Ley, P. (1979) Memory for medical information. *British J. Social and Clinical Psychology*, 18, 245–55.

Liberman, R.P. (1982) What is schizophrenia? *Schizophrenia Bulletin*, 8, 435–37.

Liberman, R.P., Wallace, C.J., Falloon, I.R.H., *et al.* (1981) Interpersonal problem solving therapy for schizophrenics and their families. *Comprehensive Psychiatry*, 22, 627–30.

Lukoff, D., Liberman, R.P. and Nuechterlein (1986) Symptom monitoring in the rehabilitation of schizophrenic patients. *Schizophrenia Bulletin*, 12, 578–603.

MacCarthy, B., Benson, J. and Brewin, C. (1986) Task motivation and problem appraisal in long-term psychiatric patients. *Psychological Medicine*, 16, 431–8.

MacMillan, J.F., Gold, A., Crow, T.J., *et al.* (1986) Expressed emotion and relapse. *British J. Psychiatry*, 148, 133–44.

McCreadie, R.G. and Phillips, K. (1988) The Nithsdale schizophrenia survey. VII: does relatives' high expressed emotion predict relapse? *British J. Psychiatry*, 152, 477–81.

McGill, C.W., Falloon, I.R.H., Boyd, J.L., *et al.* (1983) Family education intervention in the treatment of schizophrenia. *Hospital & Community Psychiatry*, 34, 934–8.

McIntyre, K., Farrell, M. and David, A. (1989) In-patient psychiatric care: the patient's view. *British J. Medical Psychology*, 62, 249–55.

Meichenbaum, D. (1985) *Stress Inoculation Training*. Pergamon, Oxford.

Meichenbaum, D. and Turk, D. (1987) *Facilitating Treatment Adherence*. Plenum, New York.

Miklowitz, D.J., Goldstein, M.J., Falloon, I.R.H., *et al.* (1984) Interactional correlates of expressed emotion in families of schizophrenics. *British J. Psychiatry*, 144, 482–7.

Miles, P. (1977) Conditions predisposing to suicide: a review. *J. Nervous and Mental Disorders*, 164, 231–46.

Moline, R.A., Singh, S., Morris, A., *et al.* (1985) Family expressed emotion and relapse in schizophrenia in 24 urban American patients. *American J. Psychiatry*, 142, 1078–81.

Nelson, A.A., Gold, B., Hutchinson, R.A., *et al.* (1975) Drug default among schizophrenic patients. *American J. Hospital Pharmacy*, 32, 1237–42.

Nuechterlein, K.H. (1987) Vulnerability models: state of the art, in *Searches for the Cause of Schizophrenia*, (eds H. Hafner, W. Gattaz and W. Jangerik) Springer-Verlag, Berlin.

Nuechterlin, K.H. and Dawson, M. (1984) A heuristic vulnerability-stress model of schizophrenic episodes. *Schizophrenia Bulletin*, 10, 300–12.

Nuechterlein, K.H., Snyder, K.S., Daeson, M.E., *et al.* (1986) Expressed emotion, fixed-dose fluphenazine decanoate maintenance, and relapse in recent onset schizophrenia. *Psychopharmacology Bulletin*, 22, 633–9.

Nuechterlein, K.H., Goldstein, M.J., Ventura, J., *et al.* (1989) Patient-environment relationships in schizophrenia: information processing, communication deviance, autonomic arousal and stressful life events. *British J. Psychiatry*, 155 (Suppl. 5), 84–9.

Ost, L.-G. (1987) Applied relaxation training: description of a coping technique and review of controlled studies, *Behaviour Research and Therapy*, 25, 397–410.

Parker, G., Johnston, P. and Hayward, L. (1988) Parental 'expressed emotion' as a predictor of schizophrenic relapse. *Archives of General Psychiatry*, 45, 800–13.

Pokorney, A. (1983) Prediction of suicide in psychiatric patients. *Archives of General Psychiatry*, 40, 249–57.

Reynolds, I. and Hoult, J. (1984) The relatives of the mentally ill: a comparative trial of community-oriented and hospital-oriented psychiatric care. *J. Nervous and Mental Disease*, 172, 480–89.

Rostworowska, M., Barbaro, B. and Cechnicki, A (1987) The influence of expressed emotion on the course of schizophrenia: a Polish replication. Poster presented at 17th Congress of the European Association for Behaviour Therapy, Amsterdam, Aug. 1987. Pub. in the abstracts.

Schooler, N.R., Levine, J., Severe, J.B., *et al.* (1980) Prevention of relapse in schizophrenia: an evaluation of fluphenazine decanoate. *Archives of General Psychiatry*, 37, 16–24.

Schwartz, A. and Goldiamond, I. (1975) *Social Casework: A Behavioural Approach*. Columbia Univ. Press, New York.

Silverstein, M.L. and Harrow, M. (1978) First-rank symptoms in the post acute schizophrenic: a follow-up study. *American J. Psychiatry*, 135, 1481–6.

Slade, P.D. and Bentall, R.P. (1988) *Sensory Deception: Towards Scientific Analysis of Hallucinations.* Croom Helm, London.

Smith, J. and Birchwood, M. (1987) Education for families with schizophrenic relatives. *British J. Psychiatry*, 150, 645–52.

Smith, J. and Birchwood, M. (1990) Relatives and patients as partners in the management of schizophrenia: the development of a service model. *British J. Psychiatry*, 156, 654–652.

Strachan, A.M. (1986) Family intervention for the rehabilitation of schizophrenia. *Schizophrenia Bulletin*, 12, 678–98.

Strachan, A.M., Goldstein, M.J. and Miklowitz, D.J. (1986a) Do relatives express expressed emotion? in *Treatment of schizophrenia: Family assessment and intervention*, (eds M.J. Goldstein, I. Hand and K. Hahlweg) Springer-Verlag, Berlin.

Strachan, A.M., Leff, J.P., Goldstein, M.J., *et al.* (1986b) Emotional attitudes and direct communication in the families of schizophrenics: a cross-national replication. *British J. Psychiatry*, 149, 279–87.

Sturgeon, D., Turpin, G., Berkowitz, R., *et al.* (1984) Psychophysiological responses of schizophrenic patients to high and low expressed emotion relatives: a follow-up study. *British J. Psychiatry*, 145, 62–9.

Subotnik, K.L. and Nuechterline, K.H. (1988) Prodromal signs and symptoms of schizophrenic relapse. *J. Abnormal Psychology*, 97, 405–12.

Tarrier, N. (1987) An investigation of residual psychotic symptoms in discharged schizophrenic patients. *British J. Clinical Psychology*, 26, 141–3.

Tarrier, N. (1991a) Familial factors in psychiatry. *Current Opinions in Psychiatry*, 4, 320–3.

Tarrier, N. (1991b) Some aspects of family interventions in schizophrenia. I: adherence with family intervention programmes. *British J. Psychiatry* (in press).

Tarrier, N. (1991c) Psychological treatment of schizophrenic symptoms, in *Schizophrenia: An Overview and Practical Handbook*, (ed D. Kavanagh) Chapman & Hall, London.

Tarrier, N. (1991d) Management and Modification of Residual Psychotic Symptoms, in *Innovations in the Psychological Management of Schizophrenia*, (eds M. Birchwood and N. Tarrier) Wiley, Chichester.

Tarrier, N. and Barrowclough, C. (1986) Providing information to relatives about schizophrenia: some comments. *British J. Psychiatry*, 149, 458–63.

Tarrier, N. and Barrowclough, C. (1987) A longitudinal psychophysiological assessment of a schizophrenic patient in relation to the expressed emotion of his relatives. *Behavioural Psychotherapy*, 15, 45–57.

Tarrier, N. and Barrowclough, C. (1990a) Mental health services and new research in England: implications for community management of schizophrenia, in *Recent Advances in Schizophrenia*, (eds A. Kales, J. Talbot and C. Stefanis) Springer-Verlag, Berlin.

Tarrier, N. and Barrowclough, C. (1990b) Family interventions. *Behavior Modification*, 14, 408–40.

Tarrier, N. and Turpin, G. (1991) Psychosocial factors, arousal and schizophrenic relapse: a review of the psychophysiological data. *British J. Psychiatry* (in press).

Tarrier, N., Vaughn, C., Lader, M.H., *et al.* (1979) Bodily reactions to people and events in schizophrenia. *Archives of General Psychiatry*, 36, 311–15.

Tarrier, N., Barrowclough, C., Vaughn, C., *et al.* (1988a) The community management of schizophrenia: a controlled trial of a behavioural intervention with families to reduce relapse. *British J. Psychiatry*, 153, 532–42.

Tarrier, N., Barrowclough, C., Porceddu, K., *et al.* (1988b) The assessment of psychophysiological reactivity to the expressed emotion of the relatives of schizophrenic families. *British J. Psychiatry*, 152, 618–24.

Tarrier, N., Barrowclough, C., Vaughn, C., *et al.* (1989) The community management of schizophrenia: a two-year follow-up of a behavioural intervention with families. *British J. Psychiatry*, 154, 625–28.

Tarrier, N., Lowson, K. and Barrowclough, C. (1991) Some aspects of family interventions in schizophrenia. II: financial considerations. *British J. Psychiatry* (in press).

Test, M.A. and Stein, L.I. (1980) Alternatives to mental hospital treatment. III: social cost. *Archives of General Psychiatry*, 37, 409–12.

Turpin, G., Tarrier, N. and Sturgeon, D. (1988) Social psychophysiology and the study of biopsychosocial models of schizophrenia, in *Social Psychophysiology: Perspectives on Theory and Clinical Application*, (ed H. Wagner) Wiley, Chichester.

Tsuang, M. (1978) Suicides in schizophrenics, manics, depressives and surgical controls: a comparison with general population suicide mortality. *Archives of General Psychiatry*, 35, 153–5.

Vaughan, K., Doyle, M., McConaghy, N., *et al.* (1991a) The relationship between relatives' expressed emotion and schizophrenic relapse: an Australian replication. *Social Psychiatry & Psychiatric Epidemiology* (in press).

Vaughan, K., Doyle, M., McConaghy, N., *et al.* (1991b) The Sydney intervention trial: a controlled trial of relatives' counselling to reduce schizophrenic relapse. *Social Psychiatry & Psychiatric Epidemiology* (in press).

Vaughn, C. (1986) Patterns of emotional response in the families of schizophrenic patients, in *Treatment of Schizophrenia: Family Assessment and Intervention*, (eds M.J. Goldstein, I. Hand and K. Hahlweg) Springer-Verlag, Berlin.

Vaughn, C.E. and Leff, J.P. (1976) The influence of family and social factors on the course of psychiatric illness. *British J. Psychiatry*, 129, 125–37.

Vaughn, C.E. and Leff, J. (1981) Patterns of emotional response in relatives of schizophrenic patients. *Schizophrenia Bulletin*, 7, 43–4.

Vaughn, C.E., Snyder, K.S., Freeman, W., *et al.* (1984) Family factors in schizophrenic relapse: a replication in California of British research on expressed emotion. *Archives of General Psychiatry*, 41, 1169–77.

Wilkinson, D.G. (1982) The suicide rate in schizophrenia. *British J. Psychiatry*, 140, 138–41.

Wing, J.T., Cooper, J.E. and Sartorius, N. (1974) *Measurement and Classification of Psychiatric Symptoms: An Instructional Manual for the PSE and Catego Program.* Cambridge Univ. Press, Cambridge.

Zubin, J. and Spring, B. (1977) Vulnerability: a new view of schozophrenia. *J. Abnormal Psychology*, 86, 103–26.

Further Reading

Bellack, A.S. (ed.) (1989) *A Clinical Guide for the Treatment of Schizophrenia*, Plenum, New York.
Useful general multi-authored text on treatment.

Birchwood, M. and Tarrier, N. (eds) (1991) *Innovations in the Psychological Management of Schizophrenia: Assessment, Treatment and Services*. Wiley, Chichester.
Up-to-date account of the developments of psychological approaches to the assessment and treatment of schizophrenia and their implications for mental health services. Includes practical advice on assessment and treatment.

Birchwood, M., Hallett, S. and Preston, M. (1988) *Schizophrenia: an Integrated Approach to Research and Treatment*. Longman, London.
An excellent general introductory text.

Falloon, I.R.H., Boyd, J.L. and McGill, C. (1984) *Family Care of Schizophrenia*. Guilford Press, New York.
A comprehensive review of schizophrenia and its treatment, with special focus on environmental and social factors. The second half of the book consists of a detailed account of behavioural family therapy as developed by Falloon and his colleagues.

Hirsch, S.R. and Leff, J.P. (1975) *Abnormalities in Parents of Schizophrenics*. Oxford Univ. Press, London.
Interesting review of early work on the relationship between schizophrenia and families.

Kales, A., Stefanis, C.N. and Talbott, J. (eds) (1990) *Recent Advances in Schizophrenia*. Springer-Verlag, New York.
Multi-authored text covering a wide range of topics, including: historical and diagnostic issues; risk factors; the treatment of schizophrenia in different countries and cultures. A heavy emphasis on biological and genetic factors.

Leff, J. and Vaughn, C. (1985) *Expressed Emotion in Families: its Significance for Mental Illness*. Guilford Press, New York.
A detailed account of the measure of Expressed Emotion and its development.

Liberman, R.P., DeRisi, W.R. and Mueser, K.T. (1989) *Social Skills Training for Psychiatric Patients*. Pergamon, New York.
A useful guide to the complementary approach of social skills training.

The following books are published reports of conferences, and include some useful, relevant, and interesting chapters.

Goldstein, M.J., Hand, I. and Hahlweg, K. (eds) (1986) *Treatment of Schizophrenia: Family Assessment and Intervention*. Springer-Verlag, Berlin.

Stierlin, H., Wynne, L.C. and Wirsching, M. (eds) (1983) *Psychosocial Intervention in Schizophrenia: An International View*. Springer-Verlag, Berlin.

Straube, E.R. and Hahlweg, K. (eds) (1990) *Schizophrenia: Concepts, Vulnerability and Intervention.* Springer-Verlag, Berlin.

Strauss, J.S., Boker, W. and Brenner, H.D. (eds) (1986) *Psychosocial Treatment of Schizophrenia: Multidimensional Concepts, Psychological, Family, and Self-Help Perspectives.* Hans Huber, Bern.

For descriptions and diagnosis readers should refer to:

American Psychiatric Association (1987) *Diagnostic and Statistical Manual of Mental Disorders (3rd ed. rev.)* Washington, DC.

Wing, J.T., Cooper, J.E. and Sartorius, N. (1974) *Measurement and Classification of Psychiatric Symptoms: an Instructional Manual for the PSE and Catego Program.* Cambridge Univ. Press, Cambridge.

For an account of medication, the following provides a useful introduction:
Lickey, M.E. and Gordon, B. (1983) *Drugs for Mental Illness.* Fremman, New York.

The following books are excellent practical guides to cognitive-behaviour therapy. Although not directed towards psychotic patients, many of these therapeutic methods are of great relevance to working with distressed, depressed, or anxious relatives and carers:

Hawton, K., Salkovskis, P.M., Kirk, J. and Clark, D.M. (1989) *Cognitive Behaviour Therapy for Psychiatric Problems.* Oxford Univ. Press, Oxford.

Blackburn, I. and Davidson, K. (1990) *Cognitive Therapy for Depression and Anxiety.* Blackwell, Oxford.

For those who are going to attempt organizational changes within mental health services, this chapter makes cautionary but essential reading:

Georgiades, N.J. and Phillimore, L. (1975) The myth of the hero-innovator and alternative strategies for organizational change, in *Behaviour Modification with the Severely Retarded.* (eds C.C. Kiernan and F.P. Woods), Associated Scientific.

Interested readers should also look at the 'Social Psychiatry and Rehabilitation' section of *Current Opinion in Psychiatry*, which provides yearly updates of relevant topics; and at issues of *Schizophrenia Bulletin*, which is a specialist journal devoted to issues relating to schizophrenia. General psychiatry and clinical psychology journals also include relevant articles as noted in the reference list.

Index